Remember
for Me

Mary Anne
Oglesby-Sutherly

REMEMBER FOR ME

ISBN 9798861806435

Editing by Dixie Phillips and ChristianEditingServices.com.

Page design by ChristianEditingServices.com.

Cover design by Rhonda Minton.

Photos courtesy of Mary Alice Lovelace Photography (www.MaryAliceLovelace.photography).

On the Cover:
(*Front cover*) Mary Anne Oglesby-Sutherly and Mrs. Florence Chatham (photo by Mary Alice Lovelace); (*Back cover*) Edwin and Ruth Marie Evans with little Mary Anne

Endorsements

"I have known Mary Anne for many years, and I have the utmost respect for her. Mary Anne has all the strengths of a true leader—she is strong in character and action. She has a strong moral character, and I believe that she has a perfect blend of knowledge, talent and people skills that is so vital to success today."

Governor Mike Huckabee

Mary Anne has been a friend for years. One of the things I love about her is her heart for people. Her heartbeat is for the people she cares for through her work on behalf of the senior adult population. I know you will enjoy her voice, but I hope you will listen to her heart.

Debra Talley
The Talleys
The Veranda Ministries Board Member

Mary Anne Oglesby is a gift to others, wrapped up with a mile-wide smile and a passion for older adults and those who care for them. With a strong "can do" attitude, Mary Anne has turned her own God-nudge into The Veranda, a ministry born of Mary Anne's compassionate heart and faithful obedience. The Veranda is a welcome respite for persons with dementia and for their Hidden Heroes, the caregivers and family members who unselfishly serve them. I know of no church that is serving this population of older adults and caregivers as well as The Veranda.

Missy Buchanan
Popular Author and Speaker
Co-Author of My Story, My Song with the late Lucimarian Roberts, mother of Robin Roberts

Mary Anne is a blessing to everyone in every setting. Her message is something powerful and honest to bless and encourage your audience.

Steve Hurst
The Steve Hurst School of Music

Mary Anne's anointed voice combined with her experience has given her the ability to relate to audiences across the country. You will truly be blessed by Mary Anne's ministry.

Gary Casto
Tribute Quartet
The Veranda Ministry Board Member

Mary Anne is one of the most thoughtful and unselfish individuals I've ever met in all my years of ministry. She has a wonderful heart for music and ministry, which is a great combination for the place God has given her to work.

Mark Trammell
The Mark Trammell Quartet

I have known Mary Anne for several years, as she has sung in our church on numerous occasions and we worked together for a local charity. Mary Anne is one of those delightful people who can light up a room with her passion for life and Jesus Christ. Her vocal performances can fill a room with electricity and engage an audience in a powerful way. I have seen her touch people in amazing ways with her ministry. I am honored to know her personally and to witness her incredible ministry.

Dr. John McKellar
Pastor, White's Chapel
United Methodist Church
Southlake, Texas

To Mama . . .

*You made a difference in my life and in the lives
of so many. You taught me how to give of myself.
You taught me how to love when I did not want to.
You taught me that love is an action word.*

*Mama, I know you are happy
beyond anything I can imagine.
I love you.*

Contents

Foreword

by Dixie Phillips

"I was hungry and you gave me something to eat, I was thirsty and you gave me something to drink, I was a stranger and you invited me in, I needed clothes and you clothed me, I was sick and you looked after me, I was in prison and you came to visit me. . . . Truly I tell you, whatever you did for one of the least of these brothers and sisters of mine, you did for me."
Matthew 25:35–36, 40

Missionaries faithfully reach out to make a difference in the lives of forgotten people groups around the globe. Mary Anne Oglesby-Sutherly from Hermitage, Tennessee, is such a missionary. She discovered an often overlooked segment of society in her own community and decided to do something about it.

Heartbroken for the neglected families of senior adults suffering with dementia or Alzheimer's, Mary Anne took a leap of faith in 2012 when she resigned from her secular job and founded The Veranda, a faith-based nonprofit ministry in Gallatin, Tennessee. At The Veranda, a primary outreach of Veranda Ministries, Executive Director Mary Anne and more than a dozen volunteers provide nurturing respite care to allow family caregivers much needed time for themselves. Services for families also include a monthly support group for caregivers and a semi-annual caregiver conference. The conference helps family members and other caregivers use biblical principles to cope with the physical and emotional toll of a stressful life situation.

The need for such services grows greater each year. Baby boomers (those born between 1946 and 1964) started turning sixty-five in 2011, and the number of older people will increase dramatically during the 2010–2030 period. The older population in 2030 is projected to be twice as large as their counterparts in 2000, growing from 35 million to 72 million and representing nearly 20 percent of the total U.S. population.[1]

People beginning to take notice of this need include some southern gospel artists who believe it's time for the faith-based community to step up and take action. Debra Talley of the Talleys serves as a member of The Veranda Board of Directors. She speaks from personal experience: "My husband's mother was diagnosed with Alzheimer's, and his father suffered with brain changes. We know firsthand what a ministry like The Veranda can mean to families like ours." The Talleys put feet to their faith by donating a portion of the proceeds from their 2015 Dove Award winning song, "Hidden Heroes," to The Veranda.

Debbie Bennett has also put feet to her faith. Debbie was married for more than twenty-five years to Roger Bennett, former pianist for the Cathedral Quartet and Legacy Five. She thrived behind the scenes as wife and mother and even co-wrote several award-winning songs with Roger. However, her most challenging role was that of caregiver during Roger's lengthy battle with leukemia, which claimed his life in 2007. Since then, Debbie has served as chairperson of The Veranda Ministries Board and volunteers wherever she can. "I've seen what the Lord can do in the lives of people society thinks have no value left. I've experienced the sheer joy that comes from ministering in this capacity. I believe God honors us when we respect those who have paved the way for us."

People outside the gospel music industry are taking notice too. Mary Malkey, the award-winning executive producer of Nashville Public Television, included The Veranda in a segment of her documentary series, *Aging Matters*. Her goal was to draw attention to the great need for faith-based institutions to be involved in meeting the needs of senior adults—and that goal seems to have been met. Mary Anne has heard from PBS stations around the country.

Mary Anne believes a health crisis is looming on the horizon and hopes The Veranda will provide a template for churches to follow. "Our present healthcare system cannot handle what is ahead. The church must address the needs of our senior adult population. I believe God has equipped the body of Christ to be on the forefront helping with this task."

Meanwhile, Mary Anne devotes herself to loving the special people God sends her way. Veranda clients have quickly become her extended family. When she married last October, female clients were her bridesmaids. Peggy, a fifty-nine-year-old client suffering from early-onset Alzheimer's, was her maid of honor, and ninety-four-year-old Florence was her flower girl. When the wedding ceremony was about to begin, Miss Edna, a Veranda client who had been fluent in French but hadn't spoken it in two years, hugged Mary Anne and whispered in her ear, "Je t'aime."

Most clients can't remember their director's name, but when they are in her presence, they never forget she loves them. Mary Anne plans to spend the rest of her life "remembering" for them and hopes others will do the same.

Remember for Me[2]

If tomorrow all my mem'ries start to fade
If familiar names and faces slip away
Would you just hold my hand
Help me understand
Remember for me

This journey we are taking will be hard
I may not say I love you but it's my heart
And though my silence will hurt
When I don't have the words
Remember for me
Remember for me

Let's hold on to the hope that will carry us through this
And cling to the faith that will help us to do this
God's arms are waiting Heaven is real
One day we'll forget this pain we feel
But until then
Remember for me
Remember for me

Remember when we held each other tight
Remember when we laughed until we cried
This is not the end
It will be that way again
Remember for me
Remember for me

Let's hold on to the hope that will carry us through this
And cling to the faith that will help us to do this
God's arms are waiting
Heaven is real
We have a promise
No disease can steal
That one day we'll forget this pain we feel
But until then
Remember for me

Preface

I love spending time on my porch.

I moved to Tennessee in 2010, not knowing where I would live or what God had in store for me, but I knew he was guiding my journey. I also knew a porch was part of the deal. I didn't bring any of my furniture, only the items I could carry in my car. People thought I was crazy, but I knew the Lord was calling me to a faith walk.

When I was a child, I often spent the night with my grandmother (Little Mama). She read to me every night and openly shared her faith with me. I remember her saying, "Mary Anne, we are to walk by faith and not by sight." Little Mama believed every Christian should take this teaching from 2 Corinthians 5:7 to heart. Her words and example shaped my small soul. It would be years before I understood exactly what Little Mama was trying to teach me, but that day did come.

Six months after I moved to Nashville, God provided me with a wonderful porch, which became my sanctuary. I met the Lord there while the doves cooed their love songs and baby birds hatched in my birdhouses. As I watched the new life come forth, I sensed God birthing something new in me. With my coffee in hand and a Bible on my lap, the Lord whispered peace to me. His presence assured me that he had everything under control. And so he did. He has opened opportunities I never thought possible.

I still take advantage of my porch every chance I get! The Lord often speaks to me during what I've come to call my Porch Time. He has guided my footsteps and led me every step of the way in the birth of a new ministry—The Veranda, a congregational respite program meeting the social, spiritual, physical, and emotional needs of older adults with Alzheimer's disease, dementia, or other debilitating medical issues.

I will share some of my faith walk with The Veranda on the following pages. Most of the accounts were written during my Porch Times as I processed my thoughts about the joys, sorrows, and challenges of each day. These are real stories about real people. Sweet people who have been dealt a terrible illness. These are their stories, not mine. I pray the stories I share will not only encourage you but also make you more sensitive to the needs of the elderly and people in your in your life, church, and community living with dementia.

Our nation is on the verge of a crisis in addressing the various needs of our senior adult population. Seniors and their families are having a hard time knowing where to turn for guidance and help. The elderly are trying to understand their purpose, and I believe the churches should be on the forefront helping with these challenges.

I strongly believe it's our Christian duty to treat our senior adults with respect and dignity. Churches should be prepared to teach their members what it means to help senior adults find and fulfill their roles in the church and in other areas of their lives. That is one of the reasons behind The Veranda. It's an honor for me to help others learn how to celebrate the blessings our seniors bring to us.

In the following pages I will introduce you to some of the members of my special family at The Veranda and share with you the many lessons they have taught me. We can all learn from people experiencing brain changes if we listen to their hearts. We need to go into their world because they can no longer come into ours.

I also hope to help you learn how to celebrate the blessings our seniors bring to our lives. I want to tip my hat to the hidden heroes in families affected by dementia. The world may have no idea what they do, but our heavenly Father sees their labor of love—and he cares.

Hidden Heroes[3]

A husband holds the hand of his bride of 50 years.
The doctor's nod confirms the sickness and his deepest fears.
He renews his wedding vows; in sickness and in health.
Faithfully he cares for her though she thinks he's someone else.

Hidden heroes are not hidden from the Father.
Hidden heroes are His special sons and daughters.
He sees them singing in the rain, loving through the pain.
Heaven knows they always bring a smile to His face.
Hidden heroes are never hidden from the Father.

Acknowledgments

To the men and women of The Veranda: Without you, there would be no program. You have been at my side, taking every step with me, for the past five years. Some thought we would never make it. On the days I was weary and wondered if I could keep going, you all stood with me. You fought the fight for me and kept me grounded. Most important, you prayed daily that God would meet our every need. Without you, there would be no book—none of these beautiful stories to share. You kept up the pace of a vigorous workweek even though you are all retired from your careers. Over 20,000 hours of volunteer time later, you are still keeping the faith. *Remember for Me* would never be if not for you. As the song says, "I will always love you." Thank you from the bottom of my heart.

Rhonda Minton: God sends friends our way during our journey on this earth. *Friend* is defined as "a person who one knows of mutual affection." Maybe that's what Mr. Webster says, but I say a true friend walks every mile with you and is there when no one else seems to care. A true friend will always have your back. A true friend lays aside personal tasks to help you even when that causes her to fall behind. I don't have enough room on this page to say how much I appreciate you and love you for your help with this book. You know every person in every story. Thank you for being my best friend in good times and bad. Thank you for all you have done to help make my dream come true. My best friend, I love you and thank you.

Julia Ellis: I would be remiss without thanking my sweet, precious, wonderful friend and second mother, Julia Ellis. One day, on a drive through Belle Meade, your home before you were "put away," you said these words: "For pity's sakes, Mary Anne, I have a friend at Vanderbilt who wrote a book about dirt. We are going to find a way to get your stories published. Us old people who drive you crazy should have stories about us. Are we not more important than dirt?" My sweet Julia, your dream for me and my dream for me are here in these pages. Without your love and selfless giving to me, there would be no book. There would be no Veranda. And even though I kept your wishes and you had no obituary and no funeral, your heart will live on in this book. Your legacy is on every page. You taught me how to really love and always remember "the old people's side" in my stories. You touched my life in a way no one else ever has. We were kindred souls on a journey. God allowed us to meet in not so good circumstances, and out of our sorrows we found peace. This book is not about dirt . . . it's about love. A kind of love I never knew until I met you at the top of the stairs on that snowy February morning . . . a divine appointment for us both.

Introduction

Statistics show that in the next twenty years, one in two people will need a caregiver. That means the other one will *be* a caregiver. Having experienced caregiving firsthand, I can tell you that the emotional, physical, and financial toll on a caregiver is staggering. Our society and, yes, the church are not prepared for what will happen in the next twenty years.

In many cultures around the world, multigenerational families live under one roof. If a family member needs care, it's done by the family in that home. Not so in our society. Many loving parents are sent to nursing homes or assisted living facilities to live out their days. Granted, there are numerous people whose circumstances make it impossible for them to care for a loved one in the home. However, many of our aging and physically or mentally challenged are warehoused for convenience. This situation is bankrupting our society, both financially and morally.

Where is the church in all this? Matthew 25:37–45 is Christ's answer to the dilemma we face. No matter what our church affiliation, we all have a responsibility to care for "the least of these."

In Nashville, Tennessee, The Veranda does just that. The Veranda's incredible volunteer staff lovingly serve the ones who need care *and* their caregivers. This book is the story of one woman's call to care for "the least of these" and her dream to make it come true.

Mary Anne Oglesby-Sutherly would prefer not to draw attention to herself, but God has chosen her to shine the spotlight on the epidemic our country is facing and the role the church must play in meeting this dire need. The seed of this dream was planted in her years ago. Then through a series of divine appointments, the beautiful soul of an elderly Southern lady, Julia Ellis, nourished that seed to fruition. Soul mates found each other and The Veranda was born.

Mary Anne left the security of a steady paycheck to step out in faith and follow the path God had set before her. Stepping out of her comfort zone and into the unknown, she has blazed a trail by developing a model for meeting the needs of our senior population that *any* church can follow.

This book is not about statistics. It's not about a program. It's about people. As you read, put yourself in these stories. Feel what these souls feel. Hear what they are desperately trying to say. If you do, you will gain a glimpse into the heart of my dear friend, Mary Anne Oglesby-Sutherly. Her heart is for people and she is a warrior for those who have no voice, people just like you and me.

Maybe in the future, it *will be* you and me.

Debra Talley
The Talleys
Veranda Ministries Board Member

Stories
from
The Veranda

After the ministry of The Veranda started, so did the stories of the men, women, and families who walked through our doors. Each one's journey is unique, yet the Alzheimer's and other brain changes drew us together on common ground. Oh, the stories I could tell. I have chosen a few of my favorite experiences—most of them journaled during my Porch Time—to share with you in this book. Be prepared to laugh and cry. You'll learn one thing for sure: ***growing old is not for cowards***.

Many thanks to the families of these special people for allowing me to share their stories.

CHAPTER 1

"Have You Lost Your Memory?"

Laughter is the best medicine. I love to laugh and have fun, don't you? I believe the scripture that tells us laughing is the best medicine, but a crushed spirit dries up the bones (Proverbs 17:22).

This week my people at The Veranda had a great time of laughing and smiling with a joyful heart. Even when a terrible disease like Alzheimer's robs them of memory, laughter creates a level playing field for all of us. Laughter is a universal language. When I laugh with someone who speaks Japanese, both of us laugh in the same language. And, oh my goodness, combining laughter with music provides a setting for a great time. This week proved that combination to be true.

It sometimes seems impossible to figure out what would make all our clients happy at the same time. But I do know this: 90 percent of them will come together for a great time when there is music. One day this week I showed a music video as music therapy for my friends. It was a video of the National Quartet Convention's *Pianorama*. Some of my personal friends are on the video, and I knew the music could be used for a sing-along. The video featured quite a variety of music styles, and there was something for everyone on there. Little did I know what a difference that one video would make to all of us.

Of course, they all loved the funny parts, especially Gerald Wolfe, the emcee. They thought he was cute. In fact, one of my clients wanted to take him home. They were particularly fond of Derrell Stewart, the "man in the red socks," as they called him. Then came a Christmas song played by Stan Whitmire, and it was amazing. Suddenly we heard twenty people singing, "Sleigh bells ring, are you listening?" The room erupted into laughter and smiles from ear to ear popped up everywhere.

They had no clue it wasn't December. They just knew that deep down in their hearts the song brought them peace and joy. They sang and sang. One little lady who never speaks "la la la'd" her way through it. It was amazing to see all the different levels of brain changes enthralled by one common theme—music. People with brain changes who restlessly get up and down, up and down out of their chairs a hundred times a day sat for ninety minutes and watched a video of people they didn't know. They didn't have to know who the people were—they heard the music. Style and performance made no difference. It was simply music, *something they could remember.* Because music is stored in a different part of the brain, those suffering with Alzheimer's or other kinds of dementia can remember songs.

One of my best friends, Josh Singletary, is on this video. He is a great guy and, might I add, has graciously made time to play for my sweet people on more than one occasion. I couldn't remember exactly where he was on the video, so I kept saying, "Okay, this is my friend Josh coming up. He is going to come play for you all one day." The next person up would not be Josh. I repeated this four or five times. The staff began laughing and teased, "We don't think there is a Josh on here."

Next person up, I said, "I think this is Josh's time." I heard a sweet little voice: "Have you lost your memory? You can't remember anything."

I cracked up laughing. Here sat a person who didn't even know what month it was asking me, "Have you lost your memory?"

Yes, laughter is the best medicine. That memory puts a smile on my face every time I think about it. You see, God knows what we need before we do. I believe that with all my heart. He knew in all his wisdom that these sweet little people needed a song that day, a song to make them smile. He also knew I needed something to make me laugh and to reflect on when my heart gets weary.

Just think, a failing brain all "tangled up" brought such laughter and joy to me. I challenge you to go look up one of these sweet people and love him or her. You will never regret it. Have you ever experienced the truth of Proverbs 17:22? "A joyful heart is good medicine" (NASB). It will be my medicine for the rest of my life.

CHAPTER 2

Je T'aime,
Miss Edner

As Valentine's Day approaches, we celebrate in fine fashion at The Veranda. We call it the "Love Day"—and for good reason. Not one staff member or volunteer will deny the valuable lessons our special friends have taught us about love. It's a special love—a love that knows no bounds. That's where my sweet Edna comes in.

I have waited almost two years to write about sweet "Miss Edner." I know her real name is Edna, but as a joke to make her smile one day, I called her "Edner." She laughed and smiled the biggest smile ever, and the name stuck. Now even her family calls her Edner. We are not making fun at all. She is so very special and deserves a special name. In fact, Edner deserves many special things, in part because she has brought us all great joy and tons of laughter. She even tried to teach us Southerners how to speak French. Now that was a hoot as we say here in the South.

A school teacher for most of her life, Edner could speak many languages and dialects. On Valentine's Day a couple of years ago we all wanted to learn how to say "I love you" in French. She was up for the challenge. Frustration is the word that comes to mind as the lesson began to wear on her. We were not very good at French. She actually told some of us just to forget it. Nevertheless, we plunged forward with great vigor. Some of us mastered it that day. We were so excited we Tennesseans could speak a little French. Ms. Edner was smiling from ear to ear. On that day, she had a purpose. She was normal for just a little while in a world that was crumbling around her. Her heart knew she was losing the ability to speak and remember all those languages she previously spoke fluently—but that day she was the teacher, and we were her students. What a great day that was.

The part of my job that hurts the most is to look back at their journey. To see how they came to us and how they are now. The great mind robber has taken its toll on sweet Edner. Another Valentine's Day has come around, and it's such a struggle for her. Do you think we would let that stop us? NO WAY! It was time for lesson number two in French. This time many things were different, but one the same—love, the greatest of all gifts. The love we have for her. Unending love for her that has brought us all such joy. Even when a person can't speak love in French or English, they can show it. They can be a vessel the Lord uses to show others about Jesus and his love. Edner taught me about love. She loves unconditionally. She loves with an agape love and no longer even understands the word. To me, that is true love.

Today was a rough day for Edner. I had never seen her cry, but today many tears fell. As I sat to chat with her, she was talking about her mother and how she was going to take a trip to see her. I could see in her eyes a longing, one I had never seen before. You see, we get to know our sweet people very well. We sometimes notice things that even the families miss. I saw a different look in those sweet eyes. My heart was quickly saddened, and I begin to try to change her mind about that trip. I could see she was upset. Looking back, I realize she wasn't upset about taking the trip. Rather, Edner was sad she would not see us while she was gone. My heart quickly told my mouth to speak positively and tell her we love her and maybe we should all go on a cruise—not to make light of her conversation but to redirect her thoughts toward something fun. She followed, but not for long. I believe she has a plan.

It was Wednesday—the day for our weekly lunch outings. Everything was great. We had a wonderful time, and Edner did well. She laughed and as always looked the menu over several times. She was trying to be herself, but I could tell that longing was still there. As we were leaving, Edner called me over and had me bend down so she could whisper something in my ear. I so wanted to burst into tears, but I could not. She gently cupped my face into her hands, tears streaming down her face, and said, "Thank you so much for helping me." My heart burst into tears, but my mouth said, "Oh, Edner, I love you and no thanks needed." Her reply? "I love you too. I really do." Those words radiated through every fiber of my soul. God had brought us together and taught us both about his love.

Most people more than likely consider Edner and others like her as non-productive, mentally unstable, and of little value or use in this world we live in. But the Lord used this little woman to stop me dead in my tracks. I had awakened this morning unhappy, tired from lack of sleep, fretting over things I couldn't change, wanting to control situations I have no control over. My day ahead was busy, really busy, doing things that in the big picture meant nothing. God sent a message to me through my sweet Edner. A message that no matter what comes my way, love is the greatest gift ever given to us. She gave me love—agape love. Alzheimer's does not restrict her love. She loves me and the staff with a heart I am not sure we can ever fully understand. Our clients show unrestricted love. What better kind of love can any of us have on this Valentine's Day?

The Bible teaches us that the greatest gift we can give someone is love. One dictionary definition of *love* is "an intense feeling of deep affection." But the Bible teaches that love is more than a feeling—it's an action. Biblical love is moral character: the way we act and treat others.

On the way home that evening, I talked to the Lord. *Please teach me to love like Edner. Let me have a heart like hers. Teach me to smile and say thank you for the kind things people do for me. Most of all, be with Edner on this journey. Help her find peace and rest for a weary body and a mind that no longer remembers the past.*

Maybe, just maybe, Edner will remember that a group of people in a respite program called The Veranda love her and always will.

Happy Valentine's Day, Ms. Edner. Je t'aime.

CHAPTER 3

From the Heart of Dixie

Nobody loves the old hymn "Blessed Assurance⁴" more than Dixie; in fact, it's her signature song. She especially loves the chorus. We all love to hear her sing, "This is my story. This is my song. Praising my Savior all the day long."

My journey with Dixie started almost two years ago. The Veranda's policy is to love our sweet people struggling with brain changes right where they are in that moment. Oh, if only those of us who are supposed to have it all together could understand what that moment is. So often we think of the next minute, day, week, or year. What if we were not promised tomorrow? What if we were not promised the next thirty seconds? How would we act or react? I am not sure I fully understand it, but I know this: Dixie taught us at The Veranda a lesson we will never forget about agape.

Ephesians 5:19 says, "[Speak] to one another with psalms, hymns, and songs from the Spirit. Sing and make music from your heart to the Lord." Dixie's song was from her heart. It went from her heart to mine and to everyone who crossed her path at The Veranda. Dixie could sing any part and even hit a high C. I was always amazed at how well she could stay on pitch. Her love for the Lord transcended a brain full of plaque and tangles.

It's a medical fact that brains shrink during this dreaded disease called Alzheimer's. Even though Dixie's brain is shrinking, her heart is not. Even during her journey through this disease, her love for Jesus is steadfast. Her ability to know where her help comes from is always the focus of her day. There is never a day she doesn't talk about the Lord.

One day we were discussing a few things as only Dixie could discuss. Alzheimer's had robbed her of nouns, and she could barely speak three words at a time. Even without the ability to speak sentences, she made the most poignant statement: "Mary Anne, you love me like Jesus does." Tears flowed down my cheeks, and I told her I could never fully love her like Jesus, but I certainly loved her from head to toe. Love radiated from her eyes, and she smiled. I am confident of this one thing: the heart that Dixie gave to the Lord many years ago was still getting messages from her Savior. I also know that Savior used Dixie to speak to all of us that day. She taught us a timeless truth. Nothing in this life can separate us from the love of God—not even Alzheimer's.

Dixie always had a way of bringing genuine smiles to our faces. The first day she came to us she was dressed in three different outfits—all different colors and styles. Her panty hose and black three-inch heels set the ensemble off. She probably dressed differently in her past world when she was an executive for a number of hospitals. She also sold real estate and was a great worker in her church, where she directed the choir.

On this particular morning Dixie was going somewhere new and wanted to look good. She put on her very best and was ready to be in charge. Those first few months she was definitely in charge! We had many long days, but trained professionals know how to get to the root of who people are. I was determined to find the sweet side of Dixie. I knew it was there and I knew the Lord would help me find her.

The brain is a fascinating piece of God's handiwork. It's like a huge filing cabinet, storing things from birth to death. We store what we see, smell, and, most of all, hear. Dixie had listened to the hymns of the church her entire life. They are stored on the right side of her brain. Her ability to reason and her memories are on the left. I knew I had to tap into the right side—God's side for Dixie. Her love for music was incredible. She recognized any song or rhythm we played for her. I quickly realized music was my way into her world. I was determined to love Dixie where she was.

Love conquers many things in life. Paul said in 1 Corinthians 13:13, "Three things will last forever—faith, hope, and love—and the greatest of these is love (NLT)." He plainly said our faith, hope, and love will last forever. That doesn't mean only until we get Alzheimer's. They will last us until we are called home. I knew Dixie's faith had been steadfast. I knew Dixie's hope was in the Lord. I also knew I could reach her through love, the greatest gift of all. She could be reached through the right side of the brain through her love for music. I knew it.

A couple of months after Dixie came to us, Debbie Bennett brought to The Veranda some of her husband Roger's music DVDs. Debbie had been Roger's caregiver during his journey with cancer. Her father had also recently died with issues from a stroke and brain changes. She knew Roger had left a legacy for her family, but I don't think either she or Roger ever thought their love of music would be a catalyst for a sweet woman named Dixie. Oh, Dixie loved that DVD. She could sing any note; no matter what key a song was in—she would find a part. It was amazing to watch. I knew this was my answer. We would talk about the Lord and the great hymns of the faith. It was my way in.

Many days when things would get a little tense, I could simply start singing, "This is my story, this is my song." Her tortured soul would immediately start to calm and that sweet voice would sing, "Praising my Savior all the day long." I knew it … she was reachable. What had always brought Dixie joy would continue to do so as long as she was on this journey called life. Nothing could or would separate her from the love of music and her Lord. Nothing.

I am not sure those who work in the world of Christian music understand how their work affects others. I am quite sure Gerald Wolf had no clue that his dream would start an Alzheimer's choir. He never knew the *Hymn Sing* video would benefit a group of sweet people in Gallatin, Tennessee, as it has. I still remember the first day I brought that video to The Veranda and played it. It was the soothing balm of Gilead. Whenever we played it, Dixie and the others would watch it and sing their hearts out. They knew all the words and even the melody. Well, Dixie knew all parts. She would even sing the bass line. She would direct the choir as they sang. She, as only she could do, would direct us all. She was back where she had started. She was directing her choir as in years past. And what a choir this was! Anyone who heard our sweet people sing in unison about the Savior who died for them would understand the love of the Father as never before. It was the most heavenly choir I have ever heard on this earth. Even when the words were all turned around and tangled up, their hearts rang out a song only the Lord could understand. You see, it's all about the heart. Dixie's heart and Dixie's song.

I have thought long and hard about how to end this chapter. I could tell you a very sad story about Dixie's journey and how she had to leave us. However, that's not how I want you to remember her. I don't want to share every gory detail about the last day she was at The Veranda. Let me just say that many tears were shed. Did Dixie understand why she was leaving? No, not one bit. She was going to a different place to live. A decision no family likes to make. But such decisions are part of the journey. It's a family disease.

I want to leave you with my sweet Dixie's words to me that day. As I told her I loved her and that the Lord would always be with her, she answered, "It will be all right! I love you and Jesus loves you!"

My sweet Dixie, I pray you never lose your song. The Bible says the Lord sings over us. I pray the Lord sings over you!

CHAPTER 4

Puppy Love

When I sit on the porch and think about this past week, I don't know where to start. What happened this week that was most important to me or to my families? What lesson have I learned that could help others with their daily walk through this journey of Alzheimer's?

I think of my special friends who have crossed my path and their journey into this darkness. It would take a lot of Porch Times to tell about them all, but I believe everything happens for a reason. There's a reason their journeys blend with my path. Some of those reasons I understand; others I am still working on.

I will start off by saying I am constantly amazed at how the mind tangled with Alzheimer's can bring such joy and sometimes peace to others. Consider this: It's a proven fact that our pets love us unconditionally. They love us no matter what. When we come in from work, they greet us—barking, wagging their tails, jumping. Ready to be loved. They have forgotten how angry they were that morning when we left them alone. How upset they were that we locked them in a room and said, "I will see you in a little while." They really don't care about the morning. They just want love and kisses right now. They want to go outside, run and do their business, and then come back in and pick up where they left off that morning—nothing that happened during the middle portion of their day counts. They just want to be loved right now. They enjoy the present moment.

That kind of puppy love is great for my friends experiencing brain changes. Puppy therapy dogs just love on them, and they love on the puppies. The give and take allows them to remember happier times. Two great ladies bring their dogs to visit my Veranda friends. We always have a great crowd for that time. They bring the dogs to brighten the lives of the clients, never expecting the dual effect the visits have had on their own lives. They find themselves overwhelmed by seeing their pets bring such joy to my sweet people.

You see, no one can come and just leave my group. My people have a way of creeping into hearts and taking up residence. I'm thinking right now of one of my sweet friends who yearns to love on someone, all the more because she knows she is crossing over to a new place. All three of those little dogs sit in her lap. I wish you could see her smile. She lets them kiss her, and she laughs and laughs. She is loved unconditionally by those furry animals.

Unconditional love. Where have we heard that before? How we all long to have that. Like my sweet friend, we yearn for it. At least I do. So do my sweet people.

The sad part is that most people are afraid to love my sweet people. I believe it's because reaching out to them forces us to face our own vulnerability. We have to admit that maybe one day, God forbid, we will be there as well. It's easier to believe that possibility doesn't exist for us if we choose not to help make the journey easier for those who have no recourse but to plunge further into the darkness. God help us when that happens because I have learned more about love from my sweet people than any other source this world has to offer. I have learned that things like money, fame, talent (or lack of it), and looks don't matter to them.

What *does* matter? This incident gives us insight into that . . .

One of the "puppy ladies" came in with a gift for my sweet little friend who loves the dogs so much because she had cried the week before. (Might I mention this "puppy lady" is married to one of the biggest country music producers in Nashville.) It was a beautiful frame holding a picture of my friend with the three puppies they bring in each week. You see, she couldn't stop thinking about how much my friend loved those little dogs. She explained to me that coming to my place was the highlight of her week. My sweet lady had touched her heart in a way she would never get over, and she had to do something for her. Well, this simple gift worked in a powerful way. That picture was worth more than gold or silver to my little friend. It has a special place in her room—right by her pillow on the bed. Yep, it brings her comfort and peace. Most of all, it is hers . . . all hers.

Do you remember the old saying "a picture is worth more than a thousand words"? I have witnessed it. It's worth more than words, money, or possessions—especially when a sweet mind can't remember what those "things" are anymore.

Hmm . . . what does that tell us? What does this say to those who believe they have all the answers but most days choose to do nothing to make a difference?

I know what it tells me. I learned a lesson this week about unconditional love—the kind of love the Lord gives us all. Maybe we should learn to give that kind of love to those who so yearn to be loved. We should spend more time loving and less time wondering who is right and who is wrong. *Unconditional*: without conditions or limitations, absolute. That's the word of the week for me.

CHAPTER 5

A Remembrance Book

"If I had a remembrance book . . ." I love that line from the show *Little House on the Prairie*. Well, if I had a remembrance book, I would enter this week as one of the hardest.

I have had several Porch Times this week. To be honest, some were filled with tears. Throughout life, we all have some days we dread. In the Alzheimer's world one of the hardest is when one spouse has to put his or her mate in a facility and then turn around and go back home. Alone. I shared such an experience with someone this week.

I must start by saying I have learned more about love, true love, from my sweet people than from anyone else in my life. This week proved to be no exception.

Psalms is my favorite book in the Bible. I love to read them, and my special friends love them because the scriptures are short and easier for them to understand than some of the longer ones. Scripture comes alive when it comes with a reality check and proof of his promises being true. Psalm 121 is my favorite, and I love the part that says God never sleeps. His eyes are always on His children. His merciful, kind, and loving eyes were on me and my sweet couple this week.

To make a long story short, on Wednesday the day all couples dread came to pass for this couple, who have been married for sixty-five years. One had to leave, and the other now faces the challenge of keeping her life as normal as possible. I had to go into their apartment and lead the husband away, away from the life he had known all those years.

For the wife, well, she had to watch me lead the love of her life down a hall and out of her sight. You see, the great robber of the mind had finally taken the love of her life away. She could no longer take care of him; his needs were greater than what she could physically address anymore.

I told her to give him a big hug; then I hugged her. As she watched from the door of her apartment, I started a walk down a path that ripped my heart out. I was taking a man, a beloved father and husband, to a new chapter of his life. A life that would never be the same. He could no longer distinguish between right and wrong, good and bad. His ability to reason—lost. Lost to a disease that had robbed him of his very being and left him wandering in a world he no longer recognized.

His loving wife watched the love of her life for sixty-five years leave her, and her present life die. Nothing would ever be the same again. Family gatherings, Christmases, birthday parties. Why? Because no matter how hard a person tries, when that separation comes with Alzheimer's, things are never the same.

She will move to a smaller place, he to a secured unit. The only sure thing I could tell her was that the great God Jehovah never sleeps; his eyes are *always* on his children.

She knows that promise is true. But will she in the dark of the night, now alone, really, truly believe and understand that God is with her? Yes, I believe she will. She believes it today too, but her heart hurts and is sad.

When I took her to see her new room, she walked around saying, "I never dreamed it would end this way. I never dreamed it would end this way." I wrapped my arms around her, and she cried. I cried. It was just plain bad, but again I said, "The great God Jehovah never sleeps; his eyes are always on his children."

On my porch I hear a mourning dove sing to me. I see a robin building a nest on the neighbor's porch. I consider all the beauty God has given us. Such turmoil in the lives of my sweet people, yet in the darkest part of the night there is hope. Why? Because Scripture tells us so: "joy comes in the morning" (Psalm 30:5).

I pray for my sweet little couple. I hope you will too. As I left work before the weekend, she approached me with a heartfelt question. "Has he asked for me?"

You see, even Alzheimer's can't stop the love of sixty-five years. I believe his heart will remember her even when his mind cannot. Why? Because the great God Jehovah never sleeps; his eyes are always on his children.

CHAPTER 6

Their Songs

It's a cool Saturday morning here. This is great porch weather. Did I tell you I have two porches now? One on the front of the house and the other one on the back.

On Mother's Day some of the ladies remembered their children. Others did not, and I was very careful not to make them feel uncomfortable about that. I took some of my ladies to the courtyard for our Bible time that day. It's always amazing to me how they can't recite John 3:16, but they can sing it. Even with their "demented" brain, as people like to say, they in some ways remember more than we do. Can you remember all the words to "Let Me Call Your Sweetheart"? How about "Silent Night"? Those "walkie talkies" (my blood boils when I hear them called that) can.

Do you know why they remember songs? Music is stored in a different section of the brain than other types of memory.

I believe the Lord made this provision for them, but I am no expert in the field. I sit here and listen to the birds singing and a train whistling in the background. I know if he hears that bird singing, he listens to my sweet people's songs—the songs of those who can't speak for themselves. They have a song only he can hear, and I believe he listens intently to them. So when you see a "walkie talkie," be very mindful that they are his children.

I love my Porch Time. When it's quiet, peaceful, and calm, I can listen better. I can hear a song meant for just me. Like right now. A mourning dove is singing a morning song to me. Can't beat it. Love my Porch Time.

CHAPTER 7

Memorial Day

As I sit here this morning, I think back on memories embedded in my mind from years ago. It's Memorial Day weekend, and everyone is celebrating the valiant men and women who have served us and helped provide us with the freedoms we have. That's what I'm doing as I sit on my porch. I have thought about this holiday all week because in my line of work, memories are a key issue framing my day.

I go to Mr. Webster's dictionary. Just what is a memory? This is his definition: "1. A person's power to remember things. 2. The power of the mind to remember."

Power is the key word in both these definitions. My sweet people have lost their power to remember. In a real way, their brain has lost its power to remember. They are powerless over what is happening to them and their mind.

As I look back over my life, I realize that without the Lord beside me, I am powerless. Many things come my way that I have no control over. I am powerless over bad memories I have stored—things I want to forget but that seem entrenched in my mind. I see some of my sweet friends also struggling with bad memories.

Just imagine you have horrible memories and get stuck in that place. During every waking minute, you relive something bad that happened to you. For example, suppose you served our country. During a battle for our freedom, your best friend was in a tank with you when the enemy threw a grenade inside. You woke up to find your friend was dead, and parts of his body were missing. If that weren't bad enough, you were so terrified that you stayed in that army tank for three days. You were finally rescued, and from that point on, things were never the same. Imagine being stuck there. I knew a sweet gentleman who was there—every day. He never got out of that tank until he crossed over, as I call it, to the point the memories no longer haunted him.

Such is this disease called Alzheimer's, the great robber of the mind. This sweet man served our country to give us freedom. He served this great country to allow me the freedom to sit on this porch, drinking coffee or sweet tea. The freedom to write about how wonderful the Lord is, remembering that when we are weak, he is strong. Jesus's grace is sufficient for all times.

That sweet little man was a true hero, one who had run the race, kept the faith, and received his reward at last. I am a much better person for having known him. Always remember, these sweet people have a story for us. They may not be able to tell it, but I am blessed because I can.

Happy Memorial Day from the porch!

CHAPTER 8

Creamed Corn Jelly

It's warmer for this Sunday morning's Porch Time. Last Sunday was cold. This crazy weather—I can never figure out what it's going to be.

Are we ever really satisfied with anything? That thought takes me back to Monday when I was on an outing with some of my sweet people.

First we had lunch at Loveless Cafe. They love it there. I always learn so much at a table watching them eat. On Monday I learned in a special way about the word perspective. I later looked it up in the dictionary just to see how many definitions of that one word I could find and how many would pertain to Alzheimer's. BINGO! Here are a few: "a view or prospect; a mental view or outlook; a way of regarding situations, facts, and judging their relative importance."

For years I have told families they should choose their battles when it comes to the care of their loved ones suffering from brain changes. On Monday, I had to put that advice to the test.

One of the sweetest little ladies I have ever known was sitting beside me. She loves Loveless biscuits just as much she loves their homemade peach preserves. She doesn't remember what happened about fifteen seconds ago but does remember her husband taking her to a restaurant for dinner. It's a place where a sweet memory and a sweet time in her life go hand in hand. Most of her day is spent wondering where she is and where she should go. At Loveless, she finds an answer. Is it reality? No, but who cares.

Okay, back to the biscuit. She put butter on the biscuit after I told her how to cut it open because she was about ready to dump everything on top. We cut the biscuit open and buttered it. Then came the preserves. She was so excited about the biscuit. She loved it!

As lunch rolled on, some of the others had to be prompted about what the butter was for. It was just so interesting for me to sit and watch the sweet, precious people who had made it to this point on their own. Soon everything will be done for them. They will no longer know what to do or how to do it.

Back to my sweet friend. She had started to eat when out came a mound of fresh hot biscuits. Her eyes lit up. "Can I have another one?"

"Well, of course you can," I assured her. It had been less than five minutes since the first one. A bowl of wonderful sweet creamed corn had been added to the table. Loveless has the best. She had eaten some of the corn and just loved it.

"Can I have more jelly for my biscuit?" she asked.

"Sure," I answered. Her spoon went into the corn.

I opened my big mouth to say, "No, that's corn," when I remembered what I always tell my families: choose your battles.

I looked at her. "Sure, go right ahead."

She looked at me and happily declared, "That's the best peach jelly I ever had. Kind of lumpy but really good!"

You see, in her mind it was sweet, thick, and lumpy. Just like the peach preserves.

Perspective? What was the definition? "A way of regarding situations, facts, and judging their relative importance."

Was it important for me to correct her? Was it worth making her feel stupid? Was it worth making her understand that life was slipping past her in fast motion with no stops along the way? No. The "jelly" was sweet and lumpy and made her happy. But most of all, it gave her a choice in a life where soon she would have no choices—only a journey into darkness, a deep darkness that breaks my heart. Remember, we must choose our battles.

Oh yeah, on the way back home from the restaurant we drove through Leiper's Fork. A little voice from the back hollered out, "Are we in Pennsylvania?"

I'll say it again. Perspective.

CHAPTER 9

War Heroes

What a great country we live in. Today is a day we all celebrate a wonderful gift given to us in many ways and with many
lives—the gift of freedom. I looked up freedom in Mr. Webster's
dictionary. Here is what he said: "the ability to act freely, release
from captivity or bondage, right to act or speak freely, right to
occupy a space, free will."

Goodness, I could do three or four Porch Times from
those definitions.

I woke up in the night thinking about what to write about
today. I have been so blessed to live in a country founded on
freedom. I am so blessed that this country was based on religious
freedom so I can serve the Lord and write about the One who
has made all this possible. He is freedom to me. He taught me
what freedom really means. How? Well, one way is my daily path,
a journey with my special friends who have Alzheimer's. This

path allows me the privilege of helping those who lose their freedom daily. They lose all those definitions listed by Mr. Webster.

My sweet friends have lost their freedom to a disease that's captured their minds. I keep a journal of sorts with names and stories just so I won't ever forget the lives I have been blessed to encounter. In my journal are several friends who served our country proudly and with honor. Today I want to tell you about two of these sweet people.

First, I was called to a home one day a few years back to assess a gentleman for a sitter. He was a WW II veteran and Navy colonel. He was a pilot, and when he retired, he taught in a flight school in Texas. I will never forget him. He had been deemed "aggressive." That word makes my blood boil sometimes. I wonder how someone using that term would feel if everything they held dear were slowing slipping away. (Okay, enough of my soapbox. That will be a Porch Time one day.)

His wife greeted me as I arrived at their home. I could tell she was worn out, but she was very gracious. She invited me in and introduced me to her husband. He smiled and saluted me. I knew I was going to like him.

We sat and "talked." Well, in Alzheimer's talk. I love it, because in their mind their words make perfect sense. He talked about flying and the war. He was so proud of his service. You see, he couldn't remember his family or anything else, but he could talk about his service to our country. Hmm, freedom—a release from captivity.

At ten o'clock the clock went off to the tune of the Navy hymn. He saluted and started singing the hymn. His eyes lit up. His face actually softened, and his words were clear. I cried then, and I cry this morning. Even the great freedom robber of the mind couldn't take that part of him away. This man who had fought to give me freedom was so proud of his service that even Alzheimer's couldn't steal that honor from him. Every hour on the hour he would sing his song and salute.

I am not sure this generation truly understands that kind of freedom. This fine gentleman has found his great reward now. On this Fourth of July, he is truly celebrating freedom. What a wonderful lesson learned about freedom. It was bought with a price, a debt I can't repay.

My sweet friends like him teach me things daily. In some small way, I can repay them for what they have done by not forgetting what they did for our country. And might I add, I can at least help make their final journey to freedom a happier, more meaningful path . . . a path with the dignity, respect, and honor they deserve. Tom Brokaw calls them "The Greatest Generation," and that they are.

It's so hard to stay on track today. So many things to say. Saying it all would take too long, so I will close with a cute story about a lady friend. She was precious and a prissy little thing, and I liked her. Her daughter would lay out her clothes every day and even put her jewelry around the hanger. She wanted everything to be perfect for her mom.

One day when I was talking to my friend, she told me about being an airplane mechanic during the wartime while her husband was flying overseas. It was so cool—a real Rosie the Riveter! You would have never guessed by looking at her all dressed up that she would have even known how to work on an airplane, but she did. I saw the pictures.

I asked her why she did it. Although by then she was well on her journey into this disease, just as clearly as you and I could speak she declared, "Well, it was the right thing to do. I had to do it for my country and for the love of my life."

The tears started flowing. Funny thing is, she didn't understand why I cried. You see, that generation did things because freedom meant everything to them. It was the right thing to do. Oh my, can we not learn so much from them?

To end our conversation, she said, "After the war, I got me a lady's job." She was beaming. I will never forget her.

Freedom, a gift given to all of us and one we should never forget—a gift given to us by special people. People whom I love and am so proud to help on their journey into true freedom. You see, I believe that one day their sweet minds will be given back to them. I believe my little Navy pilot will recover the memories he lost; he will know true freedom. I believe when my little Rosie passed, she saw the love of her life again.

To me, that is true freedom. Hope. The Bible says that people without hope will perish. I have full hope that my friends will find their freedom one day. Until then, I will love them, listen to them, and help make that journey a peaceful one.

And I will remember for them.

CHAPTER 10

"Al, Is This You Talking to Me?"

My porch is not a very cool spot to be this morning. It's humid and hot, and the bugs are driving me crazy. The flowers I have cared for all summer are fading with each passing day. No matter what I do, they wilt and their bright colors continue to fade. I find myself watering them twice a day because I don't want to them to die. I want them to keep their original bright green color and stay full of life. I don't want to see those ugly brown leaves that tell me they are withering away from this unbearable heat.

Even the plants that are supposed to thrive in the heat are withering away. Wither to me has such a sad tone to it, so I looked up its definition. According to Mr. Webster, it means this: "fade away, decay, to lose the freshness of youth, to make shrunken, dry as from lack of moisture, to lose vigor."

I read those definitions, and the first thing that came to my mind was the brain. A brain "tangled" with Alzheimer's. This is one of the hardest Porch Times for me because I personally know the family on my mind today. They are my friends, special friends. I hope and pray they know how their journey is becoming a part of my path. I hope I can write this with the respect and honor due them.

I have had the privilege of teaching at the Steve Hurst School of Music for the past several summers. It's a great week of music, new friends, old friends, and a time of renewal for me. This year was no exception. I was blessed beyond measure. You see, I believe in an odd way that Alzheimer's follows me. Why? I think because the Lord wants me to see him through them. Boy, oh boy, did I ever this year.

I have a great friend whose seventy-year-old father is suffering with "Al." That's what they call it. You see, he named it so he could speak to it. Speak to it so on those days when "Al" acts up, he can say, "Al, is this you talking to me?" A great man of God who has preached since he was eighteen had the ability to give a name to a disease that would one day consume his very being.

I have watched his progression over the last couple of years. My heart grows sad when I see him each year, but this year was different. It was a life lesson for me.

We had a great altar service one night, and I saw his daughter down front. I went to pray with her. She is hurting with a pain that can be understood only by someone who has been there.

As I hugged her neck, I was facing the back of the room. What did I see? Her dad. He was standing straight and tall, looking toward heaven with clear eyes, eyes not clouded with

Alzheimer's. Doing what? Worshiping. Praying. Thanking God for his blessings.

I just sat down and thought, "Oh, my goodness!"

He had been standing for a very long time, yet even "Al" couldn't stop his worship. I don't think I have ever been as humbled as I was that night. I was tired, weary, hungry, and thirsty, and I wanted to go to my room. Yet he was content, happy, fed, and rested. Why? Because I believe he knew his journey would take him to a place where those nights would no longer exist. He would one day not be able to stand, speak, or raise his hands to the One who has been the very source his entire life. The One he has preached about and led people to. The One who has allowed him to be a part of his mighty works.

Yes, my sweet friend knew his journey would lead him to a world of silence. But he also knew that the Lord promised him that in that journey he would never leave him nor forsake him. Even in the grip of a disease that would rob him of his mind, his heart would always be able to worship.

Can I prove that? No, but I know this: the great God Jehovah never sleeps nor slumbers; his eyes are always on his children.

As I sit here looking at my withering plants, I know Alzheimer's disease may cause a brain to wither away, literally drying up and becoming brittle just like these plants. However, we have Living Water that will never run dry. It will always quench the thirst of a heart that hurts and a soul that longs to worship the Lord. What "Al" tries to dry up will always be refreshed by Living Water.

I was forever changed by that night. My sweet friend unknowingly opened my eyes to a part of worship I had never known.

A few years have passed since then. He continues coming to the school of music each summer—and still sits in the same chair. Each year I see more signs of the disease progressing. Last year he didn't remember my name but hugged me and said, "You still sing like a bird." His wife faithfully brings him to our chapel services every night. This is a safe place for him. A place where he is welcomed each year. He is always accepted for who he is at that moment—and so he finds peace in that safe place.

What a beautiful reminder that we need to go into our loved ones' world when they can't come into ours.

CHAPTER 11

"A Pretty Woman with Brown Eyes and That Sings"

It's been awhile since I have sat down to write my Porch Time—not because I haven't been enjoying my porch, quite the contrary. The weather has been cooler, tempered by a soft gentle breeze; my ferns are much greener. I have been able to sit and watch all God's handiwork in action. Hummingbirds fighting, spiders making webs, and mosquitoes buzzing around and then enjoying their breakfast at my expense. One morning I watched two little kittens run up the neighbor's tree, fight, push each other off the branch, and then to my amazement climb right back up and start the process again. In all these frolics, one word came to mind—perseverance.

So I went to Mr. Webster to find out just what that word means. I also wanted to know how it pertains to my sweet friends, because I have learned whether having a good day or a bad one, they are always persistent. Family members caring for them are too. I have watched them persevere in an unimaginable journey with their loved ones.

Thinking about the word perseverance and what it means brings a special friend from years ago to mind—Mrs. Jewell. One experience with her is one of the funniest and best memories I have. Perseverance: "a continued effort to do or achieve something despite difficulties, failure, or opposition." Yep, that was her. She had an abundant supply of perseverance.

Some friends and I are big fans of women's basketball, and we love our basketball time. One Friday afternoon, Mrs. Jewell decided she wanted to come to a game, and we agreed to take her. At the time, she still lived at home, so we told her we would come by and pick her up before the game.

Knowing the possibility of her forgetting was great, I told her I would call early Saturday morning to give her plenty of time to get ready. She always wanted to look good from head to toe before going anywhere. Her hair was always fixed, makeup on, and her clothes ironed. She had worked her entire life and always dressed "just so." And she was not shy about anything she said. She always wanted me to date her son. Problem was, well, let's just say I would prefer someone with teeth.

Anyway, back to my story. I called her on the morning of the game, but she didn't answer. I tried a couple of times to no avail. There was nothing to do but to go on to game. The first half of the ballgame was great. We were winning. The refs were acting right. It was a terrific game.

My friends and I were chattering away at halftime, when what to my wandering eyes should appear but a little lady and a security guard coming across the court hand in hand. Yep, you guessed it: Mrs. Jewell. She was coming toward us, pointing and shaking a bony finger in my direction. I knew I was in trouble. She was angry with me. We all jumped up and ran out to meet her and the guard.

When we reached them, the guard asked, "Do you know this little lady?"

"Yes sir, we sure do," I answered.

I asked how she found us and how she got there. He told us she had taken a taxi, walked up a huge hill, found him, and all but demanded that he take her to me. However, she didn't remember my name, so she asked him to find "a pretty woman with brown eyes and that sings." Well, he had patiently walked her around the concourse until she saw us and pointed us out. The rest is history.

She watched the second half with us; then, lo and behold, three minutes before the end of the game, the announcer said, "Would Mrs. Jewell please come to the entrance of the coliseum?"

In front of everyone, we had to get up and help her climb down many steps—too many for her, but she once again persevered. Her son was there to pick her up. It seems she had called a cab to get to the game and had left a message with her son to come get her.

Perseverance! Like none I had ever experienced, and to tell you the truth, I'm not sure I have since. She came angry and left a happy, contented woman, a woman with "a continued effort to do or achieve something despite difficulties, failure, or opposition."

Remembering this story made me think of 1 Corinthians 13:6–7: "Love does not delight in evil but rejoices with the truth.

It always protects, always trusts, always hopes, always perseveres." You see, even with a devastating disease and her other debilitating medical issues, my friend trusted Jesus, she loved me, she hoped, and she was protected by his love. He helped her persevere—no matter what came.

My friends and I had a great laugh over that day's events, but more than that, we knew the Lord was trying to teach us a lesson, a life lesson that would stay with us forever.

James 1:12 states, "Blessed is the one who perseveres under trial because, having stood the test, that person will receive the crown of life that the Lord has promised to those who love him." What greater promise is there for those who go through the daily routine of caring for someone they love and watching that person slowly fade away? The Word promises that when they face trials of many kinds, their faith is tested, and when the load they carry seems more than they can bear, God will supply patience and strength in times of trial. There is hope for a better day. There is joy in the darkest hour. They can find laughter in sorrow. They can find peace in times of struggle. I guess the best way to put it is like this—there is hope!

I am not a doctor, lawyer, neurosurgeon, or senior health care expert. However, I am someone who has seen the sparkle of one lady's sweet smile, a pointing finger, and a heart of love and compassion that transcended a brain full of tangles and a diseased body to find the persistence to come be with me.

Our team won the game, but I must say, I won more sitting beside a special friend that day than I ever won watching a ballgame. This victory was so much sweeter.

CHAPTER 12

Changes

There is a tree in my neighbor's yard that I see each day—it matters not the season because it's in plain view from where I sit on my porch. It doesn't matter which end of the porch I am on or even if I am inside my house sitting in my favorite chair. I look out, and there is the tree.

It's beautiful in the spring when it's fresh and green, and it's beautiful in the fall when its leaves are bright red and orange. The best time to look at the tree is during a full moon. It's so beautiful as the moon rises over it. Whether it's summer and the branches are thick with leaves or winter when the branches are bare, the tree is breathtaking, especially with a full moon behind it.

I find solace in that tree. I watch its branches blow from side to side, and during storms I watch it bend over as if it would break. Time seems to stand still when I sit and gaze at it.

The tree goes through many changes in a year, yet most of those changes bring peace to my soul. The tree still gives me joy and makes me smile. I must admit when the storms rage, I am fearful of what might happen to it. Change—be it with a tree or with our loved ones—is hard to accept sometimes.

It's no surprise that I would look up the word change. I wanted to more fully understand its meaning. Change: "a substitution of one thing for another, to make into or become something different, to give or leave one thing for another." Hmmm, we humans do not like change very much. We surely don't like change that takes us out of our comfort zone. I know I don't.

That brings me to my sweet friends. I have always tried to put myself in their place. If I had Alzheimer's, how would I accept the changes the disease would bring to my life? How would I accept the inevitable challenges I would face?

How would I accept the fact that one day I would look into the eyes of the dearest, most precious people in my life and not know who they are? How would I accept the fact that one day I would think I was going through the bathroom door only to end up in the closet? How would I accept the fact that I would lose the ability to taste? I wouldn't know if I were eating Mexican food or mashed potatoes.

How would I accept the fact that I would forget the basic functions of using a fork, knife, or spoon? I could go on and on. I think the picture is clear. The changes are truly more than we can even begin to understand or imagine.

Now, think about this.

All these changes would lead me to a place of darkness—a place where I would know no one or even be able to think or act on my own. How would I react? I would be hurt and angry—just plain furious. I would want to lash out at someone.

That is where my special friends are.

That is their journey, and it's a long one. A journey where the only true peace to be found comes from the Lord, a family that loves them, and a special group of people who love them and their families. I know not everyone has the same calling I have—my heart is for my special friends. But I also know that the only commandment God gave Moses on Mt. Sinai with a promise attached to it was the fifth one: "Honor your father and your mother, so that you may live long in the land the LORD your God is giving you." (Exodus 20:12).

Honoring our parents is not an option from God. He requires it. As parents, we teach our children to honor and obey us. As children of aging parents, we are still expected to honor our parents, just as we teach our children to honor us. To me that means we should always love, cherish, and honor them throughout their lives no matter what changes occur as they age. Part of honoring them includes ensuring they know we love them and care. Consider these words from one of my sweet friends: "My son is very busy. He doesn't come to see me much, but that's okay. Do you think he misses me?"

Is it easy to deal with the changes? Not always. But we need to try—and to ask God for his help. This may be plain talk from a girl raised in southern Arkansas, but we must honor our parents because God says to do it, and it's just the absolute right thing to do.

Change. It's like my tree in the neighbor's yard. It goes through many changes in a year, and I find beauty with each change. Sometimes it may not be as pretty as at other times, but it's never ugly. It still makes me smile, makes me happy, and reminds me daily that the Lord God Jehovah never sleeps. Through every change, his eyes are always on his children.

Photos
from
The Veranda

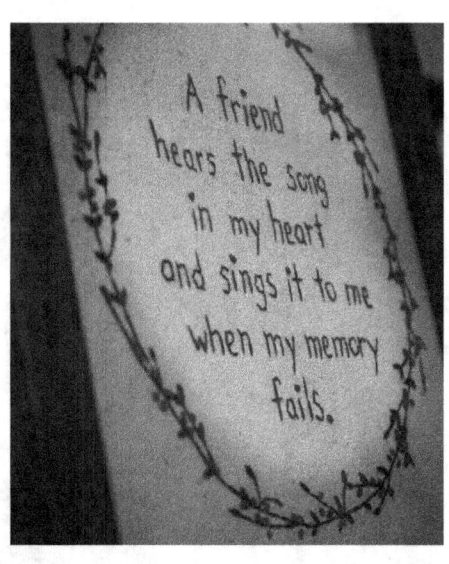

photo by Mary Alice Lovelace

A friend
hears the song
in my heart
and sings it to me
when my memory
fails.

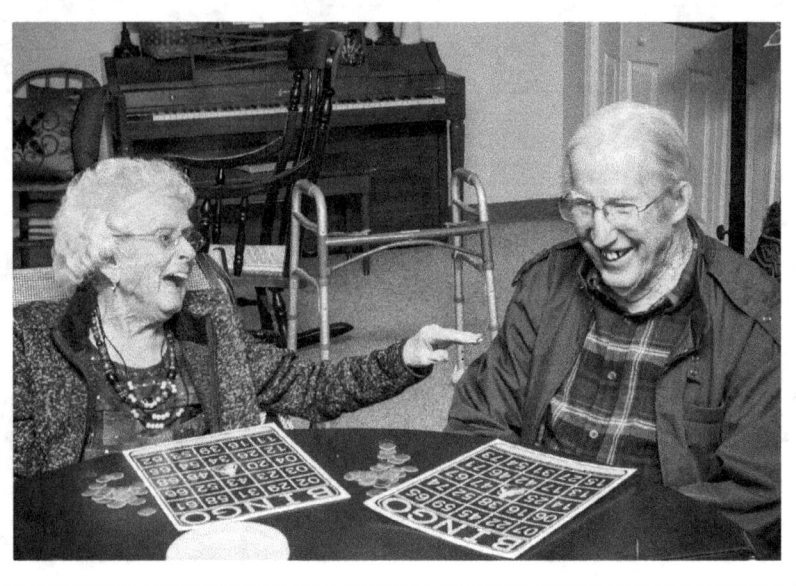

Brother James and Florence Chatham share a laugh.

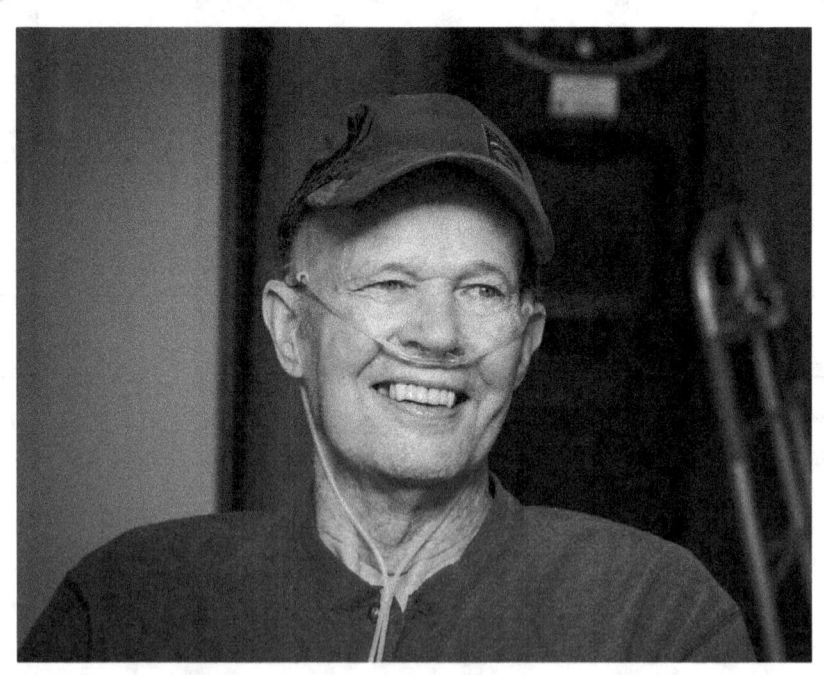

Dennis, our "Cock-a-doodle-doo!" man.

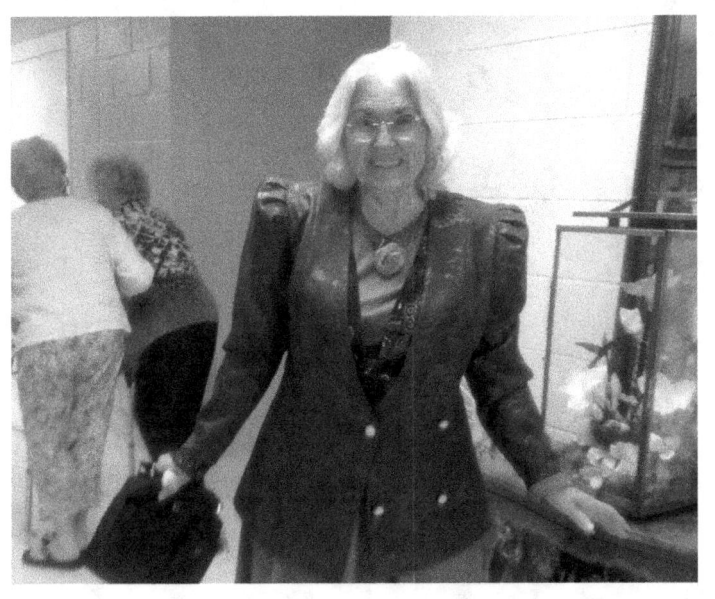

Dixie is all dressed up for her first day at The Veranda.

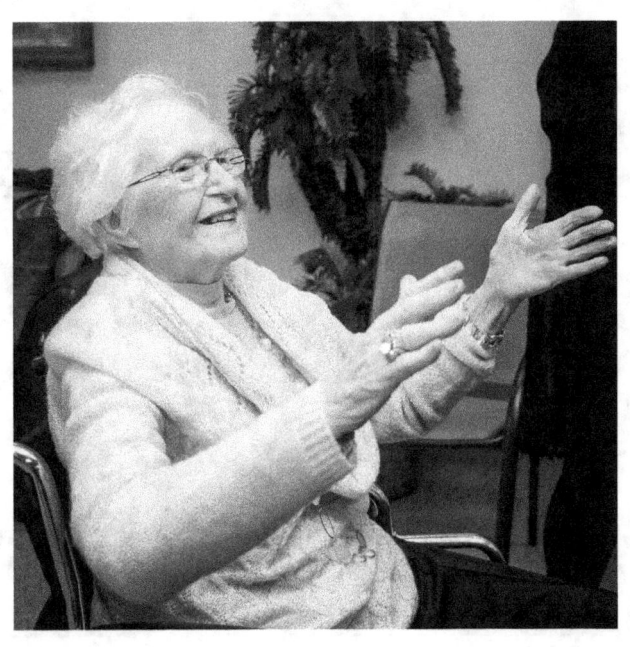

Eunice, who always "loved the Lord."

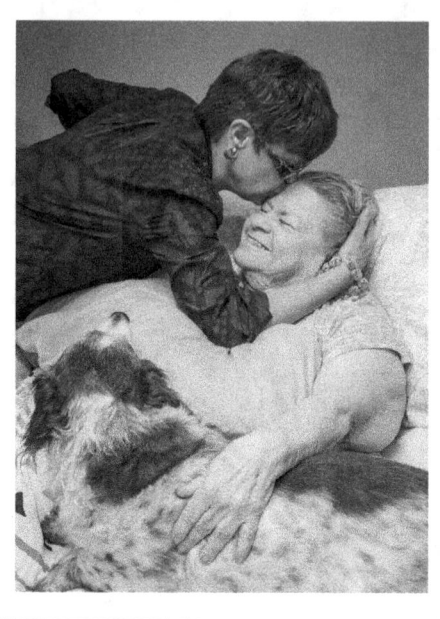

Peg greets her friend Mrs. Edna.

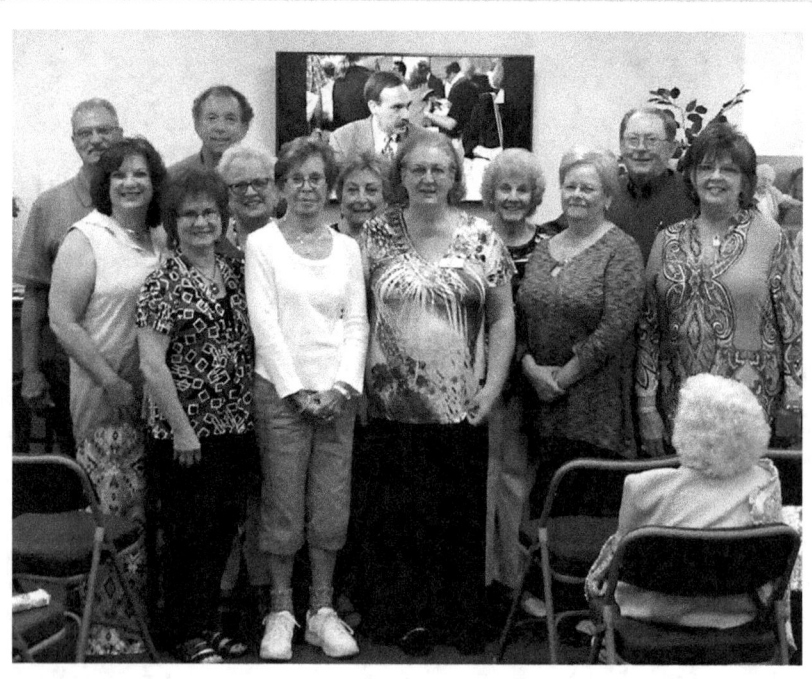

We are grateful for our wonderful volunteers at The Veranda.
They are a great example of servanthood.

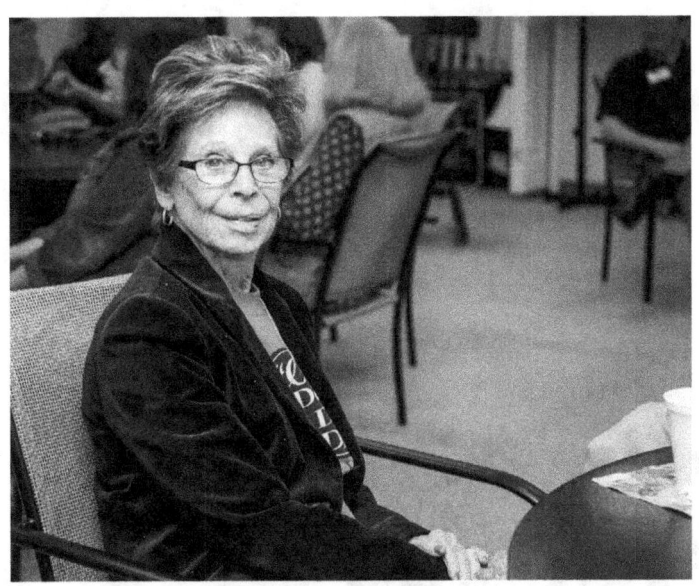

photo by Mary Alice Lovelace

Martha who started serving as a volunteer at
The Veranda, and now is a client.

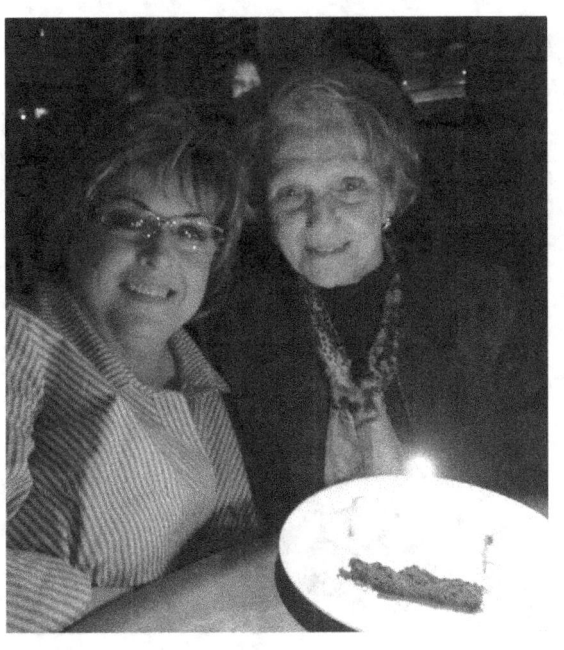

photo by Rhonda Minton

Mary Anne and Julia at a special dinner celebrating Julia's birthday.
Julia helped launch "The Project," which became Veranda Ministries.

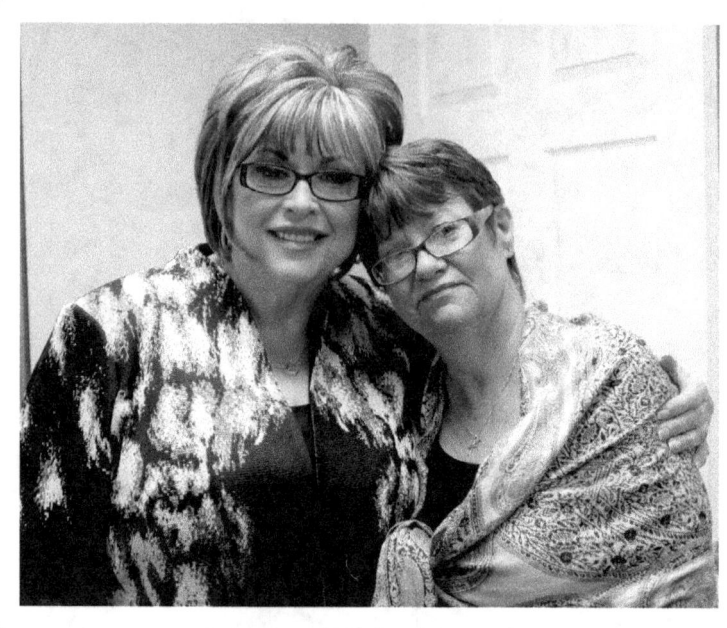

Peg served as maid-of-honor on Mary Anne's wedding day.

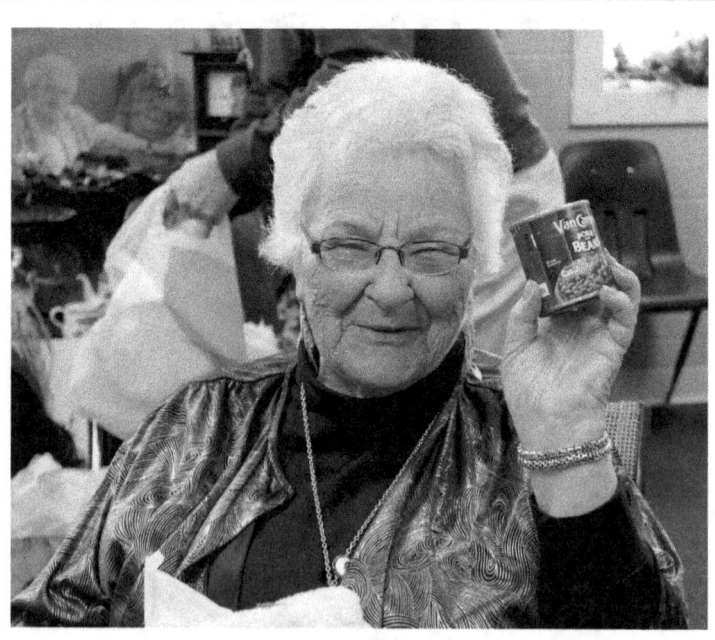

Lynn always talked about the love of her life whose leather jacket smelled good. "He smelled just like pork-n-beans."

CHAPTER 13

Scarlett, Rhett Is Waiting for You

As I sit on my porch today, we are celebrating another three-day holiday weekend, Labor Day. I love holidays for lots of reasons, but this weekend was especially nice because of a marathon weekend of The Waltons. I love that show. It reminds me so much of my family, especially my dad's side.

As I watched several episodes, many wonderful memories of my childhood came to mind. Memories of grandparents, aunts, uncles, and cousins and all the get-togethers we had over holiday weekends. Holidays at Papaw and Mamaw's house were full of laughter, food, and great tales. The stories usually centered on all the trouble my dad and his brothers had gotten into when they were growing up and the antics of their friends. I honestly think they knew everyone in Hempstead and Howard counties in Arkansas.

Growing up in southern Arkansas was a great time in my childhood. I went to a new school that had just been built in our small community. I was in the first grade the first year the school opened. It was a wonderful school. The teachers were incredible, and I believe Porch Time got its start there as they encouraged me to express my thoughts and develop my gifts.

My elementary teachers read books to us, and their stories came alive. My imagination soared. Music was also a big part of our lives as children. I sang every year at our end-of-the-year school program. One year I sang "I Love Paris in the Springtime." It was a hit! Funny, I still remember the words. Donned in a black satin evening gown, a fox stole, and high heels, I walked out on that stage just a'singin'. I think I was about eight or nine. Such great memories.

I remember friends even more clearly than all the singing. Friendships we made in that school have stood the test of time. For example, through social networking, I reconnected with one such friend (Damon Thompson), who now lives in Washington, D.C. Our friendship picked up right where we had left off—only this time we are much older. In fact, we're the same age as our teachers were when we were in that small school.

I think one reason those friendships have lasted is that we had only five to seven students in each grade. It's not hard to remember everyone in a group that small. Damon and I have had several conversations about all the great memories we have held close to our hearts. It's been just wonderful.

I also hold fond memories of friends from different times of my life. I had great times and made many friends during junior high and senior high school years. Again, social networking has become the key for everyone to get back in touch and share fond memories such as Herb's Drive-In. Herb's had the best hamburgers. I remember rushing there at lunchtime and again after school. I think it's cool that kids still do such things today.

Another wonderful memory for me is Mrs. Connie Penny, my English and journalism teacher. She instilled in me the confidence that with hard work I could be anything I wanted to be. I am heartbroken because I waited too late to tell her about my book. I never told her how much she influenced my life. So often we do the same thing with family members who mean so much to us. We wait until it is too late to say what we need to say. Regrets can devour families when this happens. I thank the Lord that I don't have that regret with my parents. However, I do with Mrs. Penny.

Recently several of us high school girls got back together. We sat out in a back yard and reminisced over all the silly things we had done like lying out in the sun until we fried, never once thinking about what all that sun could do to us. We talked about how the Lord had been good to us, how we had raised our families, and how proud we are of our kids and grandkids. Funny, we sat and discussed all those things I used to listen to as a child on Mamaw's porch during special holiday weekends. I remember rolling my eyes and thinking, "Here we go again. We're gonna hear about stealing watermelons and getting caught."

It's funny how life brings us full circle. I don't know what I enjoy more than thinking back to a happy time, a time full of joy, love, peace, and plain old fun.

I know some of you wonder what all this may have to do with Alzheimer's and my special friends. We all enjoy happy memories so much. What if you woke up one morning and everyone around you was a stranger—just a face, a face with no name. I realize it doesn't happen overnight, but it does eventually happen to people whose brain is failing.

Several of my special friends have no memory of their families, loved ones, or special friends. All their memories are gone forever. I have seen with my own eyes the sadness, despair, and heartache of loved ones who would give anything to hear one of those stories and be able to roll their eyes again at family tales. I watch tears flow down their faces because they know the stories have stopped. Family members need to learn to listen to those stories while their loved ones can still share them. They need to let go of the impulse to roll their eyes, even though they think they will scream if they hear that story one more time.

Who knows what tomorrow holds? I sure don't. But I know who holds tomorrow. I know the Lord never gives us more than we can bear. He says he will keep us to the end (1 Corinthians 1:8–9), and that means just that. The great mind robber, Alzheimer's, is no match for him. He can and will keep us safe, even on that journey.

How does this all tie together? Well, I have a story about one of my favorite special friends. She was a mess and could push every one of our buttons. I loved her and said I would probably be her in a few years. She was prissy, very Southern, and very proper. When things didn't go her way, she would come out fighting.

She never wanted to get out of the car, never. I tried everything I knew to coax her out. One morning I decided to try the Southern route. She loved movies, well, certain ones. She would watch Gone with the Wind, The Thornbirds, and North and South all the time.

"Scarlett," I said, "would you please come in? Rhett is waiting inside for you."

"Shut up, Melanie. I don't want to," she promptly replied.

This started a morning conversation theme that lasted for more than a year between two special friends, Scarlett and Melanie—just like in the movie.

When the Lord called her home, I walked into the funeral home. From the front of the room, her daughter called out, "Oh, my Melanie, Scarlett has gone home."

As tears streamed down our faces, I knew it was true. Scarlett had fought the fight, kept the faith, and, in a way not to be disrespectful, had found a much bigger and better Tara in heaven. She no longer had to be coaxed out of a car to go in—she was willing and was welcomed with open arms. I pray I will never forget her.

This one is for you, Scarlett. You are indeed one of my favorite memories.

CHAPTER 14

Sleepless in Nashville

One night I was unable to sleep. For hours I tossed and turned in my bed. I looked at my phone to see how much longer I had to endure this night, which seemed to last forever. Anxious thoughts taunted me. Recent events were still difficult for me to fathom, but they had led to this event that was all too real. We were suddenly forced to relocate The Veranda. I'll never get everything moved today! There's nothing good ahead for me, my clients, or my ministry at The Veranda. What if the weather doesn't cooperate as I try to get everything moved? How will my staff and I ever get everything done today? Endless questions poured through my mind.

I tossed and turned like a ship on a raging sea. Amid my worrying and fretting, a sweet, still, calming voice whispered, "Mary Anne, I am fully awake. I never sleep. I stay awake just so you can sleep in peace. You're being twisted up in the darkness by the evil one. He wants to block your view and give you doubts about the future. Just call out my name so I can help you."

Hopping out of bed, I hurried to my den and opened my Bible and study guide. I was comforted by the words I read: "You are surrounded by a sea of problems, but you are face to face with me, your peace."[5]

It was as if a spiritual light switch flipped on inside me. My Father had provided the weapon I needed. I just had to call on the name that is above every name to defeat the enemy. I opened my mouth and sang, "Jesus, Jesus, there is something about that name."[6]

As the Lord's presence filled the room, my focus turned to the needs of all my Veranda families who are caring for their loved ones with Alzheimer's or brain changes. I thought of how their journey was an endless 24/7 job. My one night of tossing and turning with anxious thoughts couldn't compare with their on-going exhausting days and sleepless nights. I've watched them smile through their pain and heartache. I've seen them keep their faith intact during the fire of this debilitating disease. And here I was, sitting in comfort reading my Bible and drinking my coffee in peace and quiet. I thought of my checklist of "problems" and realized I had none! No, not one! None compared with their journey.

I have always believed if we want to relieve our own stress and problems, we need to do something good for someone else, especially for someone unable to give us anything in return. We need to do it with no other motive than knowing it's the right thing to do. Jesus will take care of sleepless nights and weary days. He had certainly stepped in and fought this battle for me. He had lifted my burdens, and joy did come that morning. Thank You, Lord!

CHAPTER 15

Mrs. Eunice

I have tried to think of a clever title for my tribute to one of the most precious women I have ever had the privilege to know. I finally decided I would title this entry simply "Mrs. Eunice." She was such a rare find—a one-of-a-kind soul. Her joy was contagious, her smile infectious, and her heart for the Lord was like none I have ever witnessed.

Mrs. Eunice came to us shouting God's praises, and I know she was shouting his praises in the early morning hours when she left this world for her heavenly home. Toward the end, Alzheimer's left her unable to shout or speak on this side of heaven, but I believe her new body and a clear, untangled mind allowed her to shout her way into that place she had sung and talked about for ninety-four years.

God sometimes sends a breath of fresh air into our lives. Eunice was our breath of fresh air. From the first day she arrived at The Veranda, our hearts were cemented together with a bond of love stronger than any super glue. It didn't take long for everyone to recognize that when Eunice showed up, the party started. She spread sunshine wherever she went. Alzheimer's had stolen a lot from her, but it couldn't rob her spirit and could never sway her beliefs. Eunice knew whom she belonged to.

In Romans 10:10 the Bible states that our salvation is from the heart. If we believe that, then Eunice's brain full of tangles could not and would not stop her from loving the One she trusted the most. The Message translation says it this way: "With your whole being you embrace God setting things right, and then you say it, right out loud: 'God has set everything right between him and me.'" Eunice had set it right with her Creator many years before. It was still right the day she saw him.

There are so many stories I could write about her. However, to be honest, as I sit to write them, they become so personal that I will keep most of them to myself. However, she would be upset with me if I didn't share a couple.

One day she was singing at the top of her lungs, as only Eunice could do. "When we all get to heaven, what a day of rejoicing that will be. When we all see Jesus, we'll sing and shout the victory." Her hands in the air, she shouted, "Hallelujah! Praise the Lord!" She wasn't loud or rambunctious, but her face lit up like the morning sun. It was almost as bright as all the bling she loved so much. She had her jewelry on and her rings were as large as the fingers they graced. She often declared, "They make me shout better!"

I am not the best piano player that ever touched the ivories, but my limited skills get me by when I play for my clients at

The Veranda. You see, they don't care how well I play. They sing from a different place. They listen from a different place. It's a place of no judgment—only gratitude that someone will let them be themselves. That's what we did with Eunice. She was free to be herself with us. However, Eunice did know a good piano player. She loved "the piano man." She never called him by his real name because she couldn't remember it. She only knew that when he touched those keys, the sounds transported her to a place of peace. She didn't have the same experience when I played. One day I told her I would play for her. When I had finished one song, she walked up and said, "You're doing okay, honey." When I stopped and laughed, she blurted out, "Now get back to playing." She had a bossy streak.

We were honored to have Eunice as a client at The Veranda for four years. In that length of time people grow to love one another like their own family. Not only did we love her, but her family became our Veranda family. The day we realized Eunice's needs were greater than we could attend to at The Veranda, we were heartbroken. We assured her we would never leave her and that her Veranda family would come and see her. We kept our promise.

Less than a week ago we went to see her. Her daughter, Carolyn, called us and said Eunice wasn't doing well. I wanted to go talk to her about her journey. I knew the Lord would let me get through to her. She couldn't speak very well, but I didn't care. As I walked in, I realized her body was frail, but that sweet precious face was as content as I had ever seen. She knew she was going to take a journey. I held her hand, cried, and told her she was going to see the One she had sung about and talked about most of her life. Her face lit up. You see, that's the way God cares for us. That's the heart salvation the Bible speaks of. I began to sing her signature hymn to her: "Sing the wondrous love of Jesus. Sing His mercy and His grace. In the mansions bright and blessed He'll prepare for us a place. When we all get to . . ." Something resonated in her spirit. She responded with raised eyebrows and a smile. The joy of her life would soon call her home. She knew it and I knew it. She tried to speak, but only a few words came out. "Love. Christian. I'm sorry." Did I know in what context? No, but Eunice did and that's all that mattered.

As I looked at her in our final moments together, I was reminded of a previous conversation we had shared. "Eunice, what is the first thing you will do when you see Jesus?"

She shot back, "Well, I am not sure. I'll probably drop dead." A tangled mind, but her heart was full of love. That best describes Eunice.

Sweet Eunice, raise your hands and shout for us until we all meet up there. Save a place for your Veranda family. After all, your favorite song says, "When we ALL get to heaven."

Our hearts will be forever touched by you, but we would not keep you here a moment longer. You are free, sweet Eunice. Enjoy every moment.

CHAPTER 16

A Rare Jewel

I could not finish my manuscript until the day Mrs. Lynn said goodbye to this world and hello to her new home. There seemed to be an unending plethora of stories that flowed from her.

Oh, how she looked forward to seeing her loved ones. She often talked about being reunited with her fourteen siblings. Most of all, she longed to see her sweet husband, Keith. Many times Mrs. Lynn would have a faraway look in her eye, and I would ask what she was thinking about. She never hesitated. "I can't wait to see my husband again."

I always thought it strange that she never called him by his name but always said "my husband." Every time she mentioned him, her eyes twinkled and her face lit up like the sun. On numerous occasions I heard her say, "Oh, how I wish I could see him again. The hardest part of growing old is how much I miss him."

Their love story included raising their children and riding cross country on a motorcycle. Those of us who heard Mrs. Lynn share from her heart about her marriage realized she and Keith had a love that few people have seen or experienced.

Mrs. Lynn was a storyteller. Time does not permit me to share all her stories here. There were many and they were all fascinating. Nothing could light up a room like Mrs. Lynn sharing one of her tales. Kindness and love flowed from her heart to all of us at The Veranda. We experienced four years of Mrs. Lynn and her heartwarming stories that will last forever in our hearts.

I have tried hard to think of a word that would describe Mrs. Lynn. I considered many beautiful words, but jewel is the best. She was a very rare jewel. Mr. Webster defines a jewel this way: "a very fine example, a valued person." A synonym is showpiece. Oh my, is that ever the truth about Mary Agnes Gwythalynne Webb Mueller. She was a showpiece—just like the little red jewel box she gave me one day. Tucked inside was a note, a very special note. A note my assistant director, Libby, and I cherish. Many times Mrs. Lynn would go shopping at Goodwill. After her shopping excursions, I would find a little gift on my desk—always something with bling on it.

Just her name brought smiles to our faces. Her stories, well, let me just say no one at The Veranda will ever eat pork and beans again and not remember Mrs. Lynn. How can anyone fall in love with a man who smelled like pork and beans? Mrs. Lynn did. Who cared that the aroma came from the leather coat he wore? And what would make her hate tomatoes so much? Working as a child picking tomatoes for her family. It was part of their living, and everyone had to pitch in. If any of us couldn't understand how five kids could sleep in one bed, Mrs. Lynn explained. "Mama put three at the top and two running the opposite direction at the bottom." And she told us in great detailed how they stopped her little brother from wetting the bed. (I won't tell that part.) Most of all, her Farkle game brought joy to all of us. No one else could holler out, "My name is Mary Agnus Gwythalynne Webb Mueller and I believe I just farkled." Can you see why we think she was the best storyteller ever?

Mrs. Lynn was a proud woman. She was proud of her parents, her siblings—two of them were nuns—and her children. She was especially proud of her grandchildren. This kind of caring is not so common these days. Family is no longer what it had been when she was growing up in Springfield, Tennessee. But to Mrs. Lynn, family was everything. It was her heartbeat in the last few years of her life.

Her love for music and her relationship with the Lord were her lifelines. Her last bingo prize was a Gaither video, and you would have thought she had received pure gold. She loved watching the musicians and enjoyed all the vocal groups.

The days we had music at The Veranda, Mrs. Lynn was always front and center. "Beulah Land" would take her right to the shore where she knew Keith was. We spoke about and sang about heaven often. The truth is, Mrs. Lynn's heart was already there. She was just waiting for the Lord to call her. Her journey for the most part was over here. She knew it and we did too.

Mrs. Lynn came to The Veranda not because of brain changes like many of our clients but because she was lonesome. She did have medical issues, and as the years went by, brain changes came into play. For the most part, she wanted to be needed, to be loved, and most of all to give love to someone else. Many days she was the center of attention—but not in a selfish way. Her love toward us was pure.

We were shooting a video one day for some advertising and Mrs. Lynn agreed to be interviewed. She brought the room to dead silence when she was supposed to share in three words what The Veranda meant to her. Without hesitation she said, "It has been lifesaving to me." And as only she could say, here came these words: "Oh, I think that's more than three words." No one in that room cared. You see, she felt we were a gift to her, but she was a more precious gift to us.

Many days when I didn't know if The Veranda would succeed or if we could keep the doors open, she would walk in and announce, "I have my darling on and my go-to-hell earrings." Worries seemed to fade at that moment. Mrs. Lynn had entered the building, and I agree—she had her "darling" on.

I have tried so hard not to weep out of sadness for our sweet Mrs. Lynn. It's just so impossible not to. She was the joy in our midst. She was the joy when we could not find any. She was the one who brought hope on days when it was hard to find. She was the laughter in our hearts that kept us going. She truly was our jewel.

Mrs. Lynn's last question to Libby (our assistant director) was this: "Libby, would you save my spot at The Veranda?"

My sweet Mrs. Lynn, you will always have a spot at The Veranda. Your spirit will be with us every day. You have left eternal footprints in our souls. Your legacy of love will always be with us. Most of all, the joy you brought to our hearts will never leave us. Your spot is here, and we will hold on to your smile until we see you again.

Legacy of Love[7]
You've left us for a while.
We'll miss your lovely smile.
But death cannot erase
Sweet memories that took place

Although you've gone away
In our heart you'll always stay
Our gift from God above
Our Legacy of Love

Your Legacy of Love with us will remain,
Echoing the truths your life did proclaim.
The torch has now been passed—we raise it unashamed
Your Legacy of Love

You're with Christ above and Christ is here with me.
We're really not apart—there's just a veil between
You will always be etched in our memory
Our Legacy of Love

CHAPTER 17

Christmas Toilet Paper

When I woke up this morning and realized it was Pearl Harbor Day, memories flooded my mind. This is a very special day for me. Over the years I have had the privilege of being on the front end of care for many special people who fought hard to give us the freedoms we enjoy. My belief system has always been a vital part of who I am, and I believe God guides our paths. He is fully capable of taking my path and placing it in someone else's journey. On December 7, 2011, he placed me in a little home with a special friend and a veteran who had fought for our freedom and was now fighting for his life. He was losing the battle for himself but had helped win the war for my freedom. I was determined to help him even if it cost me the job I had at the time—which it easily could have. This man was my Christmas gift that year, and I was determined to help him in any way possible.

Mr. John was frail and lived in very poor conditions. He had no money, no heat, and very little food. Since he had no transportation, his doctor's visits were few and far between. He lived too far out in the country for any transport help from the Veteran's Administration; he was pretty much alone. He was like many others who have served our country—alone with nowhere to turn. My job was to get him help, but I knew that was not going to happen—not as quickly as he needed it. What could I do? Who could I call? Would I lose my job for exceeding my boundaries? I prayed that God would direct my path and show me who would help me. In his Word, God teaches we have not because we ask not. Well, I was asking. I also told him if he would hurry, I would appreciate it. My heart knew this man needed help quickly.

As I waited on the answer, I posted a status on Facebook about my day. I was appalled any of our veterans who fought at Pearl Harbor would be sitting in their homes going hungry. It was the Christmas season, for goodness' sake. We were celebrating the birth of our Savior, who came to set us free. How could this be? How could we as Christians not put aside our petty ways and help those who gave of themselves for our freedom?

I kept praying, "Lord, please help me." In less than five minutes I received a message from my friend Libby Perry Stuffle. She was going to the store and would meet me at the church and bring me some food. She also knew of someone who lived close to where Mr. John lived. Her name was Debbie Bennett. I knew Debbie but not well. Libby messaged her and almost immediately my phone rang. It was Debbie Bennett. Debbie and I were not best buddies at that time, but oh, what can happen when God puts a plan together—even then he was making a way for The Veranda. He was placing those special people in my path. Deb listened to my story and said, "I will go to the store in the morning and have the food ready by ten. Can I please go with you to see him?" I responded, "Absolutely!"

On December 2, 2011, I walked into Deb's house and saw not only food but also a Christmas tree, gifts to go under it, and a shirt she had bought and monogrammed: WW II Veteran. I knew Mr. John would be so grateful. I was looking at all the "pretty" things—the tree, shirts, and gifts. But we would soon learn that Mr. John would see all this quite differently. His want list was different from Deb's and mine.

As Deb and I drove up to his home, we were both so excited. You see, when you give without expecting anything in return, the joy that fills your heart is just about more than you can stand. I knocked on his door and Mr. John hollered, "Come on in." He was unable to get up from his chair that morning. We came in bearing gifts and a Christmas tree. He was so grateful but a little taken back. As only two women can do, we were chattering, loving on him, and wishing him a Merry Christmas. We told him how much we appreciated his sacrifice in the war for us. Guess what? He didn't know it was Pearl Harbor Day. We gave him his shirt and plugged in his tree. He was smiling from ear to ear. Someone cared about him and he knew it.

We unloaded all the food. I opened the refrigerator and saw there was still no food in there. I packed it full. He would have plenty of food to last for a couple of weeks. The last things we brought in were the staples: soap, paper towels, aftershave lotion, and toilet paper. We had tried to bring everything he would need. As he was watching us unload all the items, his perspective on the gifts changed Deb and me forever. He said, "Oh my! You brought toilet paper. I didn't know what I was going to do." Deb and I stopped dead in our tracks. A simple package of twelve rolls of toilet paper changed everything. Nothing brought a smile and a shout like that toilet paper. This experience totally changed our perspective. I cried, Deb cried, and Mr. John smiled. It took only toilet paper to make him happy. Christmas wasn't about cars, trucks, or any other gifts. It was about toilet paper. He had a need, and the Lord had met it.

Deb and I have spoken of Mr. John every year since. God used Libby Perry Stuffle to bring two women together who would become best friends. He already had a plan for our lives. (Deb is now chairman of the board for The Veranda.) God brought a man who was hungry and needed clothes and medical care to show us the true meaning of Christmas. It wasn't about the gifts and it wasn't even about the toilet paper for us. It was about a plan—a plan bigger than ours. A plan God had set into motion—one that would change my life forever.

The true Christmas gift to us was that we saw a need and did our best to meet that need. God looked down and said, "There you go. Learn about me this holiday season. Listen to me, and I will show you where to go and what to do. Don't worry about this little job you have. I have a bigger one for you. I will place those in your path who I know will meet your needs."

Five Christmases later I still remember Mr. John and his sweet face. He was a part of the greatest generation. He was a sweet little man who taught Deb and me one of our greatest

Christmas lessons—only in giving are we really living. Jesus said it this way, "Whatever you did for one of the least of these brothers and sisters of mine, you did for me" (Matthew 25:40).

CHAPTER 18

Flower Girl at Ninety-Four

When I got married, I decided to invite some of my sweet people to be in the wedding. One of my dear friends, Rhonda Minton, wrote this article about the wedding. Enjoy.

> Florence Chatham never dreamed when she was 94 that she would be a flower girl, but this past October she was. Florence, who suffers with Alzheimer's, was determined to make the walk down the aisle without the assistance of her walker. She hesitated once to steady her balance, and then resolutely made her way, dropping colorful autumn leaves from her hand at perfectly spaced intervals. As she rounded the last pew at the front of the church, her husband of 67 years gathered her into his arms. "I'm so proud of you, Florence."

When Mary Anne Oglesby-Sutherly, founder and director of The Veranda, a non-profit respite program in Gallatin, Tennessee, for families affected by Alzheimer's disease or other medical issues, planned her wedding day, she wanted to make sure her Veranda families were included as well.

Peggy, a 59-year-old in the relentless grip of Alzheimer's disease, served as the maid of honor. Veranda clients made up the rest of the bridal party, and each sat in the audience and held her own small flower bouquet.

Mary Anne said the wedding was a frequent topic of conversations at The Veranda and often sparked a fond memory for its clients. "I knew our Veranda family had to be part of our ceremony because it helped give them a sense of purpose and worth," she said. "For Peggy and Florence, they were not simply adults affected by brain changes on that day; they were a flower girl and a maid of honor, roles that had dignity, responsibility, and a sense of honor."

When the bride and groom entered the sanctuary, the crowd stood to greet the couple. Half of the church contained family and friends; the other half was reserved for fifteen Veranda clients and their families. As they walked up the aisle to begin the ceremony, Mary Anne stopped and hugged each client. As she hugged Miss Edna, a Veranda client who had been fluent in French but hadn't spoken it in two years, she returned Mary Anne's hug and whispered in her ear, "Je t'aime."

For those who've been around individuals with various forms of brain changes, they know to expect the unexpected. Outbursts, roaming, and other forms of erratic behavior are often the norm. However, on that special day, an entire section of dementia-riddled adults sat perfectly quiet for nearly an hour, in full attention as they watched their Mary Anne say "I do."

The guests witnessed an extraordinary day, a wedding that no one will likely experience again. Everlasting and unconditional love was on full display, as it is every day at The Veranda, where the staff cares for clients a few hours each week to allow caregiving family members much-needed respite. The Veranda is a faith-based, non-profit organization and a ministry supported by Impact Fellowship Church in Gallatin.

Most clients can't remember Mary Anne's name, but when they are in her presence, they never forget she loves them. She plans to spend the rest of her life "remembering" for them and hopes others will do the same. "If your family is one of the few untouched by Alzheimer's or illness, reach out to a family you know is affected," Mary Anne said. "You can't imagine how acts such as running an errand, making a grocery store run, or other offers can relieve a little of the family's burden."

Mary Anne encouraged people to keep in mind that sometimes the most precious things are not always new and perfect. Unconditional love—like that displayed in the Sutherly wedding and at The Veranda—can create new treasured moments that families can hold onto.

CHAPTER 19

Life through a Stained-Glass Window

As I rolled out of bed one morning this week, my eyes focused on two things: a stained-glass window and an old piano bench directly in front of it. Both items have great significance to me. They are cherished heirlooms from an old one-room church in Columbus, Arkansas. Some of my earliest memories are times spent in that sanctuary. I treasure the services that transformed my life in so many ways.

Mrs. Edna was my Sunday school teacher. She taught me about Jesus and allowed me to stand on that old piano bench and sing.

God's Word teaches this: "Train up a child in the way he should go, And when he is old he will not depart from it" (Proverbs 22:6 NKJV). I am living proof that this promise is true. My small soul was shaped for Jesus and eternity in that tiny country church. Did I sing perfectly? No, but as I belted out those hymns, I was learning a lot. The church didn't care if I performed perfectly. They cared about instilling in me a divine purpose, encouraging me to use the gifts and abilities God had given me.

God uses the simple Mrs. Ednas in all our lives. It's funny, but I can still remember during our lessons how she would touch the beads on her necklace. Oh, how they sparkled. I wanted one just like hers. I dreamed of owning a shiny necklace, standing on my stool, and singing to the rafters about Jesus.

Back then I didn't know it, but Mrs. Edna was preparing me for the way God planned to use me in the future. She saw something in me I couldn't see. She faithfully helped me hone my skills and gave me a love for music. After all, Jesus was the One who gave me the gift of song. He was the One who placed me in that tiny congregation of twenty-five people. He was the One who gave me a wonderful Sunday school teacher. And best of all, he was the One who gave me the greatest Gift of all—himself.

I am grateful for the stained-glass window to peer through every morning. It's a part of my history. Below it sits my treasured piano bench. What precious Christmases Mrs. Edna Delaney gave me! I will forever be grateful for her influence. Thank You, Lord, for giving a little girl from Arkansas a wonderful mentor like Mrs. Edna.

CHAPTER 20

Martha's Song

It's a question people often ask. "How was church today?"

My answer today has caused many tears to fall. My heart is happy and broken at the same time as I try to understand life. I just cannot wrap my mind around why the people I love have to suffer so much.

But today God gave me the answer. He is our redemption. When this world falls apart, when disease robs my sweet friends of their memory and dignity, he is their redemption and he always will be. We were made to serve the Lord. We were made to worship the Lord.

On the way to church I was trying to decide what song to sing. As I drove along listening to music, I waited for the Lord to give me a clue. Then I felt him say, "Sing song number eight."

I began to argue. "Lord, I have not sung 'When I Think About the Lord' in two years. I do not want to do it."

Well, as usual, I never win an argument with the Lord. I knew I had to sing song number eight.

When I got to church, I asked the praise team if they would help me. They looked at me as if I had two heads but reluctantly agreed. Some were grumbling but still willing. All of them were asking why we would sing a song we barely knew. I told them, "Because the Lord said so and he knows best."

Our pastor, Steve Hurst (a dear friend of mine), got there and agreed with me. He didn't understand why but knew it was the song. Even as we did our sound check, I must admit I was still wondering why we had to sing that song. The Lord spoke to me again: "Hush. Just wait and see why. I'll show you."

So that's just what I did.

As church started, I saw my sweet Martha sitting on the second row. She had come to church with two Bibles and was so proud to be there. Smiling ear to ear, she was at peace. She was where she wanted to be. Second row, second seat. Second row, first seat was empty. The former occupier of that seat, Martha's husband, was now in heaven. It was hard for me to sing and look at Martha. Her heart was so broken and her journey with Alzheimer's bleak at best, but her Savior was about to step in.

When the track started, she looked straight at me. Tears started to flow for both of us.

"When I think about the Lord, How he saved me . . . It makes me wanna shout."[8]

Martha stood to her feet, hands in the air, tears streaming down her face, and she started singing. I mean really singing. I melted. My heart was so full. Martha had her time with the Lord. His merciful heart gave Martha worship today. None of the dark journey was present. None of her sorrow was present. Just the joy that only Jesus can give.

I want to close with this. The music was wonderful today, not because of me, but because I obeyed the Lord. God wanted me to sing that song for Martha. It had nothing to do with me. It had everything to do with Martha. She came to church with a tangled brain and a grieving widow's heart. She needed that song. The funny thing is that I needed it too. God knew that, but I was stubborn and wanted to do things my way. I wanted to sing the song I wanted, but God in his mercy spoke to my heart. I'm so thankful I listened.

Lesson learned. All of us who sing and work in ministry need to be very careful. When we murmur and complain, God hears us. I could be in Martha's shoes one day. Trying to hold on to the life I know and love. I could wake up one day and not even know where I am or who I am. Most of all, I could be in a journey where I can't worship. Not able to attend church. But today I saw worship straight from the throne room. A tangled mind worshiping a Savior whom she accepted, a Savior who has promised he will never leave her.

By the way, she stood through the entire song twice. Hmmm, we complain if we have to stand, but for Martha it was a privilege.

A good Sunday. Yes, it was. Good for me and, most of all, good for my sweet Martha.

CHAPTER 21

A Coat of Love

We have heard many times about the coat of many colors. First, of course, was the beautiful coat of many colors Joseph's father gave him (Genesis 37). Dolly Parton wrote a song, a book, and even made a movie about her special coat of many colors—which, by the way, was absolutely amazing. Dolly loved her coat so much. She didn't care what anyone else said. Her coat was a special gift—a gift of love.

Many times in my ministry the Lord allows my heart to hear his voice. I heard his voice loud and clear this week. Although my coat story is quite different from Dolly's, it still centers around a coat, a coat wrapped in love.

The Bible says this in John 15:13: "Greater love has no one than this: to lay down one's life for one's friends." I know this scripture isn't written about a coat, but it is written about the love God gives us for our friends. It's a kind of love that allows us to look past our worldly possessions. It's the kind of love that helped one of our Veranda volunteers look past the value of a piece of fabric for the love of a friend—a friend who had just gone into a place you and I would not understand unless we had a failing brain.

I have wrestled on how to even write what happened, but this story is so poignant and powerful, it must be shared. My special friend was taken to a deeper place of mental fear that we "healthy-minded" people will never understand. A paralyzing fear gripped her very being. She in an instant was taken to a new part of a journey she knows will eventually be her demise.

Have you ever thought about waking up in the morning and not knowing who you are, where you are, what day it is, or what time it is? My sweet friend lives it every day. She will say, "Please remember that for me. I am having trouble. What day is this? Where is my car? Who brought me here? Where am I?" The next day the questions start all over again. That's where she is.

On the day of my story, the fear of wearing those awful "diapers" everyone talks about became a reality for her. She knew by what had happened that she had slipped a little. She was crying, shaking, clinging to me. I cried with her. My heart was broken too. Truth is, one of her fears was coming to pass. She knew it and I knew it.

She had wet her pants.

For the first time she had no control over the flow. Worst of all, her friends knew it. We were there and saw it happen. Did it bother us? No, not for the reason she was thinking. It bothered us because it was one step further into her journey into brain changes. You see, true friends empathize and feel each other's pain. True friends lift each other up. True friends talk about how they themselves have wet their pants. True friends laugh it off. And most of all, true friends find a way to lessen the pain. As true friends, we did just that.

God guides each of us on our journey. That day he sent a message to one of her friends (a Veranda volunteer) about a coat—a simple new coat made of fabric, thread, zippers, and a few buttons. That coat was used for a divine purpose. Her friend put that coat on the seat of her car because my special friend refused to get in the car with her wet pants and ruin the seats. What a beautiful expression of love from this friend who sacrificed something of her own for someone in great need. I listened to her say, "You can sit on my coat on the way home. Oh, don't you worry about my coat. It was going to the cleaners in the morning anyway. Just sit right down on it."

Guess what? My special friend did just that. Hopped right up in that car and sat down on that coat. Did it change what had happened? No, but it did show a sacrifice—a sacrifice of love— by someone who loved a friend more than a worldly object. Someone who realized people and their feelings are far more important than "stuff." This is love at its finest moment. Love from the heart of a caring friend, love that transcends a disease called Alzheimer's. God's Word is true. Nothing can separate us from his love, not even a tangled brain ravaged with Alzheimer's.

I spoke with my volunteer later that day to see how everything went as she got our special friend settled back in her home. She said it was good. If you don't read anything else I have written, please pay attention to this: My special friend had said, "Thank you so much for letting me use your coat. I don't know what I would do without you or Mary Anne."

That's why we do what we do. That thank you money can't buy. That thank you took courage. That thank you was an admission that she had reached another place in her journey—one that takes her closer home. Is she scared? Yes, but not of death—just scared of the journey.

If I could beg, I would, but let me just leave you with this. As Christians and members of the church of Jesus Christ, we must learn to lay our coats down to help those who can't help themselves. Why? "Not all of us can do great things. But we can do small things with great love."[9] Let us learn to love more. Let us learn to be better friends. Friends who will lay down our coats for others.

CHAPTER 22

"Peace, Mary Anne"

It has been a year since my sweet mama went to heaven. So many emotions are going through me. A year It doesn't seem possible. My thoughts go to the horrendous series of events that lead to her death . . .

Mama's last month on this earth was a journey our family will never forget. A journey of medical horrors and confusion. A journey in which three kids demonstrated their unconditional love for their mother by struggling to find answers in the chaos and doing all they could to care for her.

There is no timeline for grief. There is no easy way around it. You have to walk right smack dab in the middle of it to get through. It took me a year to get the courage to share the story I have penned for you. Many times during that year I have thought about how to say what my heart knew had to be said.

I've heard people say, "There is a silver lining in every dark cloud." Maybe that's true, but it's hard to find sometimes.

I repeatedly hit the rewind and played buttons in the recorder of my mind, asking the Lord to show me how to see any kind of good in a horribly sad deed. My only answer was to tell the truth. The Bible says the truth will set you free. Sharing our family's story to help others is freeing for me. I pray our devastating experience will help guide another family whose loved one is in the care of others. I pray they will read this and speak up for their loved one who has no voice. Family members must be their aging relative's advocate, or that loved one may spiral downward into a compassionless abyss.

In our present broken medical world, we are not given many choices. Professionals tell us what to do. After all, they have the degrees and credentials to know what is best for our loved ones. Mama's generation believed that without wavering. If an educated doctor said it, then it was the gospel truth. But we need to remember that even doctors are human. Some are caring individuals who do their best to help. Others may not care so much. And some may not be as skilled as we might think.

Please understand I am not bashing doctors or the medical field. I am merely telling you our family's horrific experience. We lived through a nightmare. I wish I could say what we experienced is a rare incident, but I am afraid it isn't. Your family could be next, so listen well to what I am about to tell you and do everything you can to ensure nothing like this happens to your loved ones. I want to share this story in Mama's honor, hoping maybe someone will read it and find help in making the right decisions.

We could see that Mama's medical condition was declining. Her heart disease, diabetes, neuropathy, and vascular brain changes were getting worse. Her choices were sometimes not the best, but we wanted her to live at home as long as she could. My sister and brother were wonderful to her. We had all been taught that children are to take care of their parents. Mama had taken care of hers, and we three children had watched that. Now we were ready to do the same for her.

Our nightmare began on February 4, 2016. We never dreamed our lives would change forever that day. Mama had an appointment with her podiatrist for a procedure to remove part of a bone—purportedly a simple process. He had done a similar procedure on her about six months earlier. In preparation for that first procedure, we had stepped in and asked, "Do you know our mama is a heart patient and is on blood thinner?" Apparently they didn't. Had they not checked her medical history? They stopped the procedure and followed protocol on removing her from blood thinner. She tolerated the first procedure fairly well. Now the doctor had decided to take some more bone off another part of the same foot. His decision turned out to be deadly mistake.

Once again, they forgot about the blood thinner. They not only failed to make sure Mama was off the blood thinner before her February appointment but also did the "small" procedure in the office. When my sister retrieved Mama after the procedure, she was shocked when she saw the sink in the examining room—it looked like a bloodbath.

Following this second procedure, the bleeding continued throughout the night and all the next day. We called the doctor's office to see if they had taken Mama off her blood thinner meds. The nurse's response? "Oh, my gosh! We flat forgot."

Our nightmare continued unfolding. That day in February our mama ceased to exist as we knew her. She was sent home with pain pills, and we were told not to unwrap her foot. The situation was complicated by the fact that Mama was insulin dependent and had severe neuropathy. My sister called me because Mama's foot was bleeding profusely and infection was beginning to set in. On Saturday, February 6, Mama passed out, and we called 911 for an ambulance. The foot was still bleeding.

For the next month, my mama was pushed from one hospital to another. During her stay in a nursing home, she had a heart attack, and we finally ended up in a hospital in Little Rock, Arkansas. At least there we knew her cardiologist, and he would tell us the truth. However, by the time Mama got to Little Rock, we all knew she was headed to her heavenly home. Mama's frail little body was eaten up with infection, and her heart was worn out. The onset of hopelessness hit us like a ton of bricks.

"There's nothing more we can do for her." My sister blinked back the tears and asked, "How long does she have?" The doctor replied, "Maybe three months." Mama lasted only five days.

As in most families, some of the children live near and others live away. I was the one who lived away. The urgent call came on Saturday night, February 27. "You need to get home immediately." When I had received calls about Mama's illnesses in the past, I would pack up and go, and Mama would always rally. This time was different. Early the next morning I headed to Arkansas, crying the entire trip. I felt a gamut of emotions—anger, sadness, frustration. Mile after mile I pleaded with the Lord to please let her be the same mother I had always known. He graciously granted my request.

I walked through the door, and there she was, sitting straight up in her red recliner. I went to her and told her how much I loved her. For the next few hours we had a precious visit. We spoke of things we had never talked about before—things my heart will always treasure. I really believe Mama knew she was going home, and she had some things she needed to say before she left. After our visit, things fell apart. I knew she wasn't going to be with us much longer. Instead of asking God to keep her here, I prayed, "Please don't let her suffer any more."

I'm not sure how we lived through that Sunday to Monday. We knew why Mama was in this bad shape. It could have been prevented, but the horrific deed was done and couldn't be changed. Life handed us a terrible blow, and we as Ruth Evans' children did what we had always been taught to do. My mother's instructions had always been clear: "Do what I tell you to do." And so we supported her wishes in letting her go.

As the children of aging parents, we should do as they ask rather than what we want. I have told many family members that it's not about what you want, but what your mom or dad wants. Ask them how they want to leave this world and then follow their wishes. No second-guessing, and no "I am going to do what I want to do."

We are all so happy at the birth of a child. It's so exciting to be a part of a new life. But how much happier does it make us to know when loved ones close their eyes to this family that they will see Jesus and the family on the other side? Yes, we as children of aging parents should step back and think about "minding" our parents as we did when we were children. In Deuteronomy 5:16, God instructs us to honor our fathers and mothers. He didn't place a timeline on that instruction that releases us once we are adults. We should listen and heed their wishes. When they say it's time—it's time.

It wasn't about us children last year on February 29. It was about my sweet mama and what she wanted. As her children, we did just that. We held her hand, told her how much we loved her . . . and to heaven she went. I believe we loved her right into the arms of Jesus. The last words she and I exchanged were expressions of love.

"I love you, Mama."

"I love you too."

After she passed, I had to figure out how to keep from becoming so bitter that I would be useless to comfort my family. During my darkest hour, God whispered these words of hope to me: "Use Mama's story to help others."

Never have I ever been more determined to be an advocate for those in situations similar to Mama's.

Never have I ever been more determined to see the wrongs made right for those living with brain changes.

Never have I ever been more determined to believe that someone out there will listen to me when I say, "I beg you to check it out."

Check out all the facilities and medical team. Assisted living facilities, nursing homes, hospitals, and doctors. Check out all the drugs your loved ones are given. Be their advocate. If you can't, find someone who can.

If you feel your loved one is being abused in a community setting, check it out. It's your right. You pay the bills. That is your loved one's home. The community staffers are not your boss—you are theirs. Ask lots of questions.

Ask questions when a doctor says, "It's a simple procedure." I promise you that with Mama's diagnosis, nothing was simple for her. Simple procedures can cause severe complications. If something like this can happen to me, it can happen to you. I know the right questions to ask. I know what to look for, but I never saw this coming. I was completely blindsided.

The year following Mama's passing was confusing and painful for our family, but we have found peace. Was it easy? No. There were times I wanted to hit a few medical personnel. How dare they tell me I was too close to the situation to be objective? How dare a hospital tell us to take Mama home because there was nothing really that wrong? I could go on, but I won't. I think you get the picture.

Daddy had left this world because of complications from taking Vioxx. My siblings and I lost both parents because of a medical system that let us down. It's just the truth. I wasn't even sure it was possible to forgive and find the sunshine in this awful ordeal until one day I was looking at family pictures. I saw Mama and Daddy standing in front of a church with stained glass windows on Easter Sunday. That same window is casting hues on the desk where I'm sitting to write this story. You see, Jesus truly is in control. He was in control that February—and he is still. If anyone knows Mama was wronged, it is the Lord. He fights the battles, my friends, and he always wins. He will never lose. And no matter what happens, if we trust him, he will bring good from it.

There have been times I have second-guessed myself, questions rolling through my mind: "Did I do the right thing? Did all of us do the right thing?" We were handed a situation we did not ask for, nor did my sweet mama. How do you make a badly done medical procedure right? I can't, but God can and did when he spoke those sweet gentle words to me: "Peace, Mary Anne." I now have peace and can help others like Mama and Daddy. Someone needs to stand up and be an advocate for our elderly. It may as well be you and me.

No matter what happens on this earth, we are promised a home not made with hands. Mama and Daddy are both whole, together in heaven with Jesus. No brain changes, no diabetes, no heart issues, no mangled foot, and no pain or sorrow. I found the silver lining. Truth will always win.

"When God has another plan. Walk on and just say 'Yes.'"[10] As I sang these words at Mama's funeral, I knew we must always remember that his plan is best.

CHAPTER 23

The Greatest Gift

This question was asked in a great Christmas movie I watched this weekend: "What was the first Christmas gift?" Throughout the entire movie, one of the key actors tried to figure out the answer. He assumed it was love. However, he was told that was partially correct but there was more. The movie continued, and at the end he realized that the real meaning of Christmas centers about a baby, a special baby who would save the world and teach us about love. Jesus was the first Christmas gift—and the greatest gift of all time. He brought the world a love that people still do not comprehend. To be honest, I am not sure we mortals can understand such a perfect gift of love. That's Mary Anne theology.

Love is a gift given to us in many ways from the Lord. We see love extended to us from a manger and a cross. Mr. Webster defines love as "an intense feeling of deep affection." Mary knew that deep affection toward her sweet baby boy would one day become an intense feeling of sorrow. She knew she would have to give up the one she loved with all her heart. I believe Mary struggled with that as any mother would; after all, she was human. Deep inside, Mary knew her sweet little boy would willingly give his life in a true act of love toward anyone who has ever lived or ever will—even those who deny him. Mary knew Jesus was the greatest gift ever given.

Anyhow, the movie was great and ended as a good Christmas movie should. The trouble is, for some families, real life isn't a Hallmark movie. That is certainly true for my sweet Veranda families. However, there are Hallmark moments in their journey, and that's what I want everyone to hear about.

As the staff of The Veranda, we are determined to make Christmastime as close to a Hallmark moment as we can. It's not always easy but always so worth the effort. One day this past week we were sitting in The Veranda discussing world events. To some that may sound funny, but, oh, do we have some great discussions! We had just read our morning devotion, and I asked the clients to share about one of the greatest gifts they had ever received at Christmas. I knew there would be all kinds of answers, but never expected one particular response we received. I am not sure any of us will ever be the same after that Thursday morning.

As soon as I asked the question, one of our clients, Brother James, quickly said, "That sweet lady over there." He pointed across the room at his dear wife. Oh, my goodness, her face beamed with a smile that lit up the room. You see, the great robber of the mind has crept into a wonderful love story that has lasted for sixty-eight years. It was almost prophetic to me. The line that Alzheimer's draws in families was clearly drawn in our little room. She on one side of the room, and he on the other. Life forever changed by the dreaded "A" word. When it invades a family's life, Christmases are never the same. Life is never the same. But that evil mind robber can't stop the heart. In Brother James's heart was a love I am not sure this generation will ever understand. It's a love that survived World War II, a love that survived thousands of miles between them, and a love that to this day puts an ever-present smile on both their faces. Both are ninety-three years old and they still hold hands, still want to be together, and still have each other's back. Their journey on this earth was for their family and for serving that little baby born to save us all from our sins. You see, he is the key to their love.

Brother James met Mrs. Florence at church two days before he was to leave for the war. He was stationed in New Guinea for 1,037 days. They never really had a date, at least not like we think of dates today. However, she wrote to him and he wrote to her. It was a love story that would forever change my heart and the hearts of others in The Veranda that day. You see, Mrs. Florence kept all those letters. Yes, all 937 of them. They are tucked away in an old suitcase. A suitcase of love—true love, a love that transcends time and all the heartaches of this world.

I don't think there was a dry eye in the room. This beautiful picture of love was a Christmas gift to me and to everyone else in the room. Oh, how I wish we as Christians could have that kind of love for one another. I know Brother James and Mrs. Florence have a different kind of love, but we all could learn from it. We could be more like the Lord wants us to be. How wonderful to be the hands and feet of Jesus in a world trying its best to destroy Christmas by taking the very giver of love and life out of it.

This couple has served the Lord their entire lives. What a gift for their family! There is no need for gifts in boxes and pretty paper for them. You see, the gift they have given to their children is not available for a price. The gift is a life serving the Lord and being wonderful godly parents. The gift is living an example of true love that the family can hold on to when the great mind robber tries to destroy their lives. That sweet family will sit down to a wonderful Christmas dinner, look across the table at their parents, and truly celebrate the gift of Christmas. When the time comes that all families dread and their mama or daddy doesn't remember them, this family will be able to look past the failing brain and straight into the heart and still see love.

Our Christian lives are centered on the heart. How many times have we been told, "It's not about the mind. It's a heart issue"? We accept the Lord in our hearts. If we truly believe that, then even when the mind can't remember—and in their case, when Florence doesn't remember James—her heart will always love and know him. I truly believe that. I also believe nothing can separate us from the love of the Lord. It's a heart issue. This might be Mary Anne theology, but I believe it! There is no greater Christmas gift than the love of a Savior for his people. No greater gift than the love of two people that has spanned sixty-eight years and a world war. No greater gift than the love parents have for their children. No greater gift than children loving their parents. I could go on and on.

Although it's not a Christmas carol, "What the World Needs Now" is one of my favorite songs about love. "What the world needs now is love, sweet love. It's the only thing that there's just too little of. What the world needs now is love, sweet love. No, not just for some but for everyone."[11] May we at this Christmas season learn to give the gift of love. I am so thankful for everyone who has loved on The Veranda this year. We are truly blessed, and we wish you all a very Merry Christmas filled with his love!

[**Postscript**] Since I journaled this entry, Mrs. Florence has passed away. As a family, her loved ones agreed to let her go out on her terms. She literally quit eating and drinking. Her husband stayed by her side the entire time. Even in the end, their special love conquered Alzheimer's—they still knew each other.

CHAPTER 24

The Power of a Song

On numerous occasions I have told my families connected with The Veranda that the heart is where we find peace. When their loved ones have brain changes, the heart and soul still march on. How do I know this? I have witnessed it.

I received a powerful video clip recently from a family walking through the challenges of a loved one experiencing brain changes. It confirmed to me just how much power there can be in a song. How do I know this power is real? Because the Lord has taken me there too. More than once. And I've learned that when he gives a song, he will never take it back. Even when people can no longer speak, I've seen them sing words to songs they sang earlier in life.

A piano stool in my bedroom is my go-to place when I need to hear from the Lord. There are a few favorite books on it and a plaque above it that reads simply faith. Sitting on my bed near the stool, I can look out the window and see cows and turkeys. Most of all, I enjoy watching the breeze blowing and the listening to birds singing. This is my space of peace. The Lord visits me there—and he speaks to my heart.

The Shepherd of my soul gives my heart a melody as I listen to his handiwork. As I sit there on the side of my bed, he teaches me the power of a song. I find peace there. My mind goes back to when I stood on that same stool to sing as a child. I can close my eyes and see a little girl singing, "When upon life's billows we are tempest tossed. When you are discouraged thinking all is lost. Count your many blessings, name them one by one. And it will surprise you what the Lord has done."[12] So many memories flood my soul through the lyrics of that timeless hymn.

The power of a song stirs my heart and always transports me to a peaceful place. I have often observed how it does the same thing for my clients who are experiencing brain changes. In fact, they may not even talk anymore—but I've heard them sing hymns from long ago. How can that be? How can someone with a brain disease that robs them of memory remember all those lyrics? Music is stored in a different part of the brain than other memories. Please know I am not a doctor; I am not an expert on Alzheimer's. I have no degree in theology, but this one thing I know. His Word says in Philippians 1:6 (NASB), "For I am confident of this very thing, that He who began a good work in you will perfect it until the day of Christ Jesus." In other words, he abides in the heart. No matter what happens in the brain, Jesus is ever present in the heart. And that heart still holds the song.

The video clip I mentioned filled my heart with joy. It came from a family I had been working with for several months through the difficult journey of their mother's brain changes. So many things had been going wrong, and they were not in a good place. They had been facing many difficult questions: What do we do? What is best for our mother? How do we know what Mama would want? Too many people were providing inaccurate information while the family was trying their best to do the right thing. Their hearts were broken, and their minds were weary.

When they asked, "What do we do now?" I always answered, "What would your mama want?" I never asked what they wanted but always turned their attention to what they felt their mother would want. How would she want to live her final days in this world? Would she want her life prolonged by machines?

We need to talk with our loved ones before they are diagnosed with Alzheimer's or another kind of dementia. We should be proactive in finding out their desires and make sure we do our best to fulfill those wishes. This wonderful family determined to follow the course they thought their mother would want. Then, in their already difficult journey, their mother took a turn for the worse.

Jesus stepped in to give them hope as only he can do. The video clip showed how a simple hymn caused a voiced silenced by this dreaded disease to awaken and sing about a Savior she still knows. He still brings a song to her heart. The family had gathered around her bed to sing familiar hymns. My client had been a soul-winner and won many souls to the Lord. Music was her joy. She could remember very little and had not spoken clearly in a few days, but the Lord gave them a gift—the power of a song. Her memory had failed her, but the song lived on. Her spirit recognized whom she needed. Her soul that had started a good work was still there. The Lord camped out on her bed and gave this family hope, peace, and joy as their beloved mother joined them in song—singing harmony! He was carrying on the good work in her. She had a message for all her family on that day: "I need Thee, oh, I need Thee; every hour I need Thee; Oh, bless me now, my Savior, I come to Thee."[13]

So many times I tell my families that the heart is where we find peace. Even when our loved ones have brain changes, their soul marches on. How do I know this? I have witnessed it. This sweet family witnessed it too. One day soon their mother will go to Jesus. It doesn't get better than that. And on that day, her song will still live on.

CHAPTER 25

Words of Hope—
and a Challenge

My favorite Scripture fills me with hope—hope for my special people . . . hope for their families . . . hope for all of us caring for them. "I lift up my eyes to the mountains—where does my help come from? My help comes from the LORD, the Maker of heaven and earth. . . . The LORD will keep you from all harm—he will watch over your life; the LORD will watch over your coming and going both now and forevermore" (Psalm 121:1–2, 7–8).

What does this psalm mean for my sweet people? It means hope and assurance in God's promises, all through both the day and night. He made everything. The great God Jehovah is all powerful, and an all-powerful God stays awake to make sure his children are protected. Nothing and no one can deter him from protecting his own. That is a promise and a comfort I hold on to for my sweet people. He will watch over them, keep them safe, give them peace when they are afraid, and surround them with people who will love them.

Some seasons of life are difficult to understand. We must trust that, as the psalmist said, God indeed watches over his children. He watches over me, and I know he watches over my sweet people and their families.

People experiencing brain changes love with a special kind of love. People who are frail and can't take care of themselves, well, they are trusting. They trust that people in positions of authority will do as they have promised. Is that true? Sometimes—but not always. Please, if you have loved ones in the care of someone else, be very careful, be very watchful, and always know "all that glitters is not gold."

I pray that this book will help families prepare for their journey with their loved ones experiencing brain changes. I pray that the stories I share will encourage them not to give up. Families who have loved ones in communities now. Families who are taking care of loved ones at home. I understand the challenges as they walk with their loved ones on a journey into the world of aging. Whether that journey is a happy one or one that leads us into a world of tangles, darkness, and eventual death, aging is a journey all of us will experience.

My greatest desire has always been to help those who are lost in the maze of healthcare, Medicare, and worst of all, poverty, to be afforded the same luxuries as those who can be placed and cared for without worry. I know a family that pays nearly $80,000 a year for home care for their parents. Few can afford to do that. And how about Alzheimer's medicine—and other medicines—that are not generic? Some medicines are so expensive people have to do without them. Consider all the people in the United States who can't afford thousands of dollars a month to care for their loved ones. And those who find it difficult, if not impossible, to get help for loved ones who are aggressive, hard to manage, stay up all night, and, to be blunt, use the restroom anywhere and everywhere they want to. What happens to them? Sometimes it is easier not to think about these issues because deep down, thinking about them makes us face our own mortality.

Churches are full of hurting people trying to manage their lives and the lives of their loved ones.

Okay, church, just what and where is our mission field? Is it in the shadow of the steeple? How are you going to help the families who have a loved one suffering with brain changes and have no support? Will you be the hands and feet of Jesus in your corner of the world? Will you provide Bible studies or services for people experiencing brain changes and their families? Teaching at their level? Singing the old hymns they love? Will you visit them and love on them? Will you help families with the challenges?

As you read my last Porch Time story about one of my sweet people named Peg, I hope you will be motivated to let love prevail and reach out to others. What can you as an individual do to make a difference? What can your church do?

God has given each of you a gift from his great variety of spiritual gifts. Use them well to serve one another. Do you have the gift of speaking? Then speak as though God himself were speaking through you. Do you have the gift of helping others? Do it with all the strength and energy that God supplies. Then everything you do will bring glory to God through Jesus Christ. All glory and power to him forever and ever! Amen. (1 Peter 4:10–11 NLT)

CHAPTER 26

Peg's Gift of Love

I grew up in rural Arkansas. I remember being taught this valuable lesson there—love always wins. My grandmother told me about a Savior who would sustain me in times of good and bad. Why? Because he loves me. And he wants me to share that love with others.

The Bible teaches God is love. First Corinthians 13:4–7 describes godly love beautifully: "Love is patient, love is kind. It does not envy, it does not boast, it is not proud. It does not dishonor others, it is not self-seeking, it is not easily angered, it keeps no record of wrongs. Love does not delight in evil but rejoices with the truth. It always protects, always trusts, always hopes, always perseveres."

I observed this kind of love in action demonstrated by a sweet friend named Peg in a very special way at The Veranda. My people at The Veranda never cease to amaze me when it comes to love. They love in a different way than we "normal" people do. Peg taught my staff of volunteers and me a lesson about love that we will never forget.

We were blessed to have Peg with us. She was a wonderful young woman who was fifty-seven years old. Yes, too soon to be diagnosed with early onset dementia—but that's what had happened. Peg and I were the same age. We were both single and loved to do girlie things. We both wanted the chance to date. But Peg had one major problem—brain changes.

On her first visit to The Veranda, I could tell she was very uneasy. She was surrounded by people twenty years older than she was. They had nothing in common. She wanted the beach and sun. They wanted to sit in a rocking chair and be left alone. Peg felt too young for The Veranda, but brain changes level the playing field. The disease process makes its victims kindred spirits. But in this case, although Peg shared the others' symptoms, her desires were totally different from theirs.

Her sister was in desperate need of some respite time, and Peg needed to be needed. We had to figure out a way Peg could stay at The Veranda and be happy. Peg wanted to work and make money. She wanted to be self-sufficient. We figured out how to make that happen. I would "hire" Peg, and she would be in charge of loving on the other clients—a job she was willing to do and was good at. Every Friday her sister would bring me an envelope with money in it. I would hide the envelope in my desk and when the week was over, I would call Peg into my office and pay her. I wish you could have seen her beam.

The first thing I noticed about Peg was her authentic love for our sweet people. She loved them with all her heart. She knew how to shower love on them in ways that most of us "normal" people don't seem to get. She was far enough into the disease that there was no "oh, those people are crazy." But there was a battle raging inside Peg—one she is still fighting today. Who am I? What is happening to me? No one knew better than Peg. In the dark of the night, she would lie in bed not able to sleep—she knew her life was changing. But she also knew that God was on her side.

Peg had a very troubled childhood—one most could not even conceive. On-going abuse and neglect made Peg a teenager and young adult with many issues. And her past would come back to haunt her again later in life. That time was nearing. But above all this, she had a great capacity for love. She knew how to receive love and had no problem giving love. It was and still is an amazing thing to watch.

Peg loved her job. She worked hard "loving on her people" as she would say. You would find her kissing them on the cheek and bringing them food. She was our hostess. But Peg had a purpose in a world that was slipping away from her.

One Tuesday as I was doing paperwork, a text came in from her sister. We had been talking all about love the week before for our "News and Views" portion of the day. Something must have clicked that day with Peg. She had gone home and talked with her sister. Peg had changed her mind about her job. She did not want to be paid anymore. She told her sister, "Please tell Mary Anne I can no longer take money for my job. I want her to use it for those sweet people I take care of." Being paid and feeling self-sufficient had been so important for Peg. But serving by loving had become even more important. That is First Corinthians kind of love.

No matter how you slice the pie, that is true love. Love from a tangled mind beginning to fade away. Love from someone who had endured an abusive childhood. Truthfully, my sweet Peg never had a chance. Life was never good to her. But no matter what her circumstances, Peg had grown to the point where love prevailed.

The most special gift Peg gave me was an understanding of true, unselfish love. She was willing to give up what was so important to her for a group of people she did not know by name but knew by love.

God shows us love in many ways. This time it came to me in the form of a woman named Peg. I loved her so, and we had such a bond I was determined to include her in my wedding. I asked her to be my maid of honor. Of course, I had to explain what that meant. The look on her face when I asked meant the world to me. I honestly didn't care that much about me the day of the wedding. It was Peg's day to shine. God smiled down on us that day. Peg walked down the aisle with her bouquet. She stood at the front with her flowers, and I will always believe that on that day Peg knew she was loved. She told her sister, "I wish Mary Anne was my mama." Those were the sweetest words I had ever heard.

Even though brain changes had taken most of her mind, Peg still recognized love. She knew I loved her that day, and I will always remember the love lesson she taught me.

It's all about love. Jesus's love for us. Our love for him—and for one another. Love never fails.

Afterword

I praise God for the many ways he is working through The Veranda to touch people's lives. The words below are from a client's daughter, an example of the letters I often receive. Each one is a testimony of God's love.

Finding The Veranda for my father was like finding shelter in the middle of a storm. I had so many unanswered questions and no one to answer them, not even the doctors or nurses. I needed a break, not a break from my father but a break from his horrible disease that robbed us both. I was frustrated and so was he. Little did I know, my lack of knowledge and approach were causing the frustrations we both endured.

The day I walked through the doors at The Veranda with my father, I met Mary Anne. She was kind, warm, and knowledgeable. She welcomed us as if she had always known us. She invited my father to stay and I told her there was no way he would get that far away from me. Right before my eyes, she gently guided him to fellowship with other seniors. She sat and spoke with me about the disease and taught me more in that hour than any doctor or nurse had ever mentioned to me before. She gave me resources, knowledge, and a break. She watched over him so I could run errands, and he enjoyed it so much. I left out those doors that day with a whole new attitude. I left confident, strong, and determined that I could and I would take care of my father. With her mentoring me, I was able to relieve a lot of stress off my father, which was caused by his disease. There are tools and tips in dealing with a person with Alzheimer's, and Mary Anne did not fail to share it all with me.

The Veranda is not just a gathering place for the elderly; it is clearly a ministry and is led by a woman with passion and love for anyone who walks through those doors. I can't imagine what life would have been like for my father or myself during that time had I not gone to The Veranda that day.

Shenah Mangrum

Notes

[1]"Older Americans 2016: Key Indicators of Well-Being." Aging Stats: agingstats.gov.

[2]"Remember for Me." © 2017 Gordon Mote, Dixie Phillips, Sue Smith; New Haven Records (BMI); Asheville Music Publishing (BMI); Chris White Publishing (BMI); Universal Music - Capitol CMG; Songs from Bobb Avenue /WillyDot Music (BMI). Lyrics used by permission.

[3]"Hidden Heroes." © 2015 Dixie Phillips, Sharon Phillips; Asheville Music Publishing (BMI); Chris White Publishing (BMI). Lyrics used by permission.

[4]Frances J. Crosby, "Blessed Assurance." Public Domain. Timeless Truths: http://library.timelesstruths.org/music/Blessed_Assurance/ (April 27, 2017).

[5]Sarah Young, "Jesus Calling: Enjoying Peace in His Presence," January 15, 2016. *This Ministry That We Share:* http://myemail. constantcontact.com/This-Ministry-That-We-Share---January-15--2016. html?soid=1115218628364&aid=vui8jLQ4wgw (April 27, 2017).

[6]Bill Gaither, Gloria Gaither, "There's Something About That Name," © 1970 William J. Gaither.

[7]Dixie Phillips, "Legacy of Love," © 2000 Paxie Music. Lyrics used by permission.

[8]James Huey, "When I Think About the Lord," Copyright© 1998 CFN Music. *Worship Song:* http://www.worshipsong.com/songs/songdetails/when-i -think-about-the-lord (April 11, 2017).

[9]"The following quotes are significantly paraphrased versions or personal interpretations of statements Mother Teresa made; they are not her authentic words." *Mother Teresa of Calcutta Center:* http://www.motherteresa.org/08 _info/Quotesf.html (April 12, 2017).

[10]Daryl Williams, "When God Has Another Plan." *PraiseCharts:* https:// www.praisecharts.com/songs/details/22517/when-god-has-another-plan-sheet -music/ (April 12, 2017).

[11]Lyrics by Hal David; music by Burt Bacharach, "What the World Needs Now." Released 1965. *SongFacts.com:* http://www.songfacts.com/detail .php?id=3820 (April 13, 2017).

[12]Johnson Oatman, Jr, "Count Your Blessings." Public Domain. *Timeless Truths:* http://library.timelesstruths.org/music/Count_Your_Blessings/ (April 14, 2017).

[13]Annie S. Hawks and Robert Lowry, "I Need Thee Every Hour." Public Domain. *Timeless Truths:* http://library.timelesstruths.org/music/I_Need _Thee_Every_Hour/ (April 14, 2017).

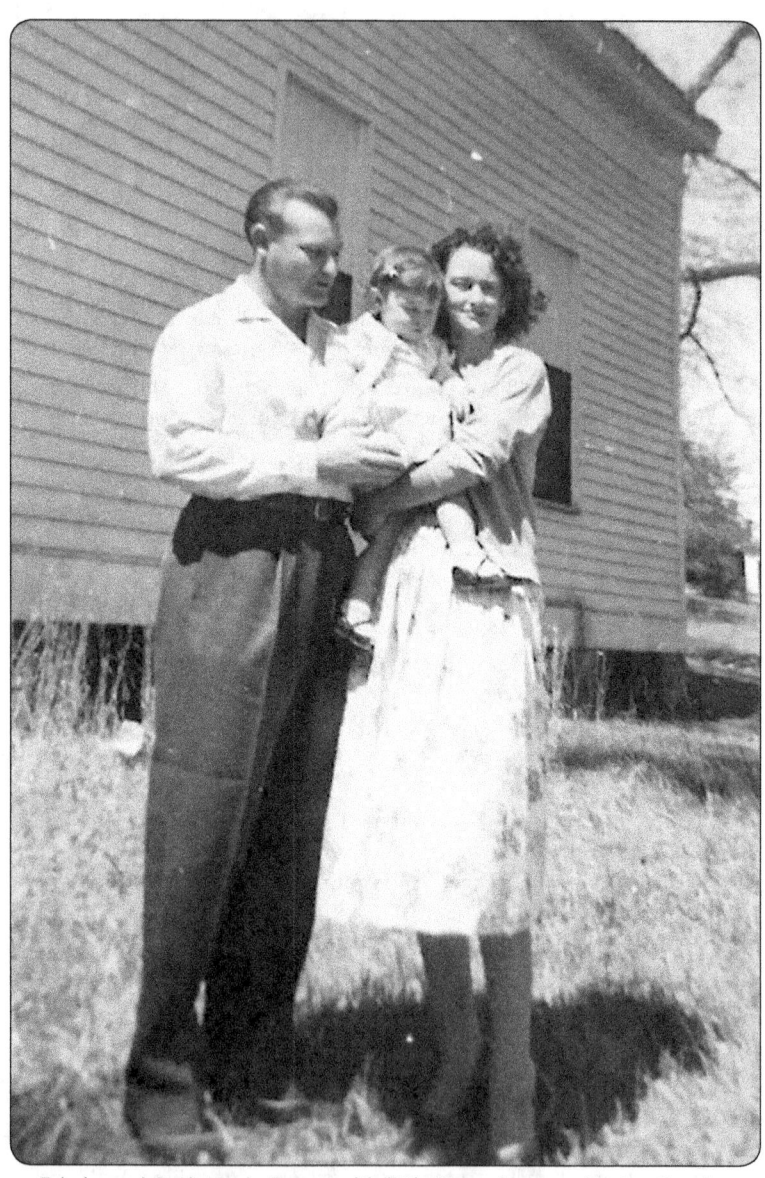

Edwin and Ruth Marie Evans with little Mary Anne on Easter Sunday outside the little country church in Columbus, Ark.